THE CANNABIS

GROW BIBLE

Growing Marijuana For Beginners How to Grow Marijuana Indoor & Outdoor, The Definitive Guide - Step by Step, Cannabis Strains

ANDERIA ZETTA ANDREW PAULL

TABLE OF CONTENTS

INTRODUCTION

—————————— ◆ ◇ ◆ ——————————

First off, I would like to thank you for choosing this book. I hope that you find it helpful and informative.

No matter what you call it, marijuana, cannabis, pot, or weed, it has a long history of human use. For ancient cultures, they didn't use marijuana to simply get high, but, instead, used it as herbal medicine. This likely started in Asia around 500 BC. America's history of cannabis dates back to the early colonists who grew it for textiles and rope.

In this book, we are going to cover how you can grow cannabis. First, we will go over the life cycle of cannabis. This will look at every single change that the plant goes through before it can be harvested.

Then we will look at the various strains of cannabis. This will cover how to spot the difference between Sativa and Indica, and we'll explore 12 varieties of weed and the effects they have.

Next, we will move into getting your seeds ready for planting and growing. For the most part, the germination process will involve soaking the seeds in water for some length of time. After that, you will be able to plant them.

Next up will be looking at the vegetative growth stage of the cannabis plant. This will take an in-depth look at what to expect during this stage, as well as what your plants are going to need from you and mother nature at this time.

After that, we will discuss the process of cloning. Cloning is a very popular process if you want to have a cannabis plant growing at all times. As you will find out, you don't want you to have a male plant around, so cloning is the next best way to start another plant.

Then we will move into the flowering stage of life. This is the part we have all been waiting for, but it's not ready to harvest just yet. Here we will look at what your plants will need from you to make sure they grow the best buds.

The next two chapters will look at the harvesting, drying, and curing process. This is probably the most important part and is something that you can't skip over. It will seem like a long wait, but it will be worth it.

Then we will go over how to grow your plants indoors. Over the next three chapters, we will look at the different aspects of having an inside cannabis garden and what you will need to grow healthy plants

Next, we will cover how to grow cannabis outside. This brings with it the problems of unpredictable weather and pests. Don't worry, though; we will go over that as well.

Lastly, we will wrap things up by talking about how to breed your plants. This is similar to the cloning process but is slightly more advance. Don't worry, you don't have to breed your plants if you don't want to, but it is interesting to learn about.

Let's get started.

CHAPTER 1

THE LIFE CYCLE OF CANNABIS

———————————— ◆ ◇ ◆ ————————————

It can be rather confusing when you start growing marijuana, especially when you have no idea what to expect. You think you have been doing everything just right, but when you harvest, you don't get as much as you thought you would. Maybe you need to learn a bit more about the life cycle of cannabis so you will be able to grow the best crop possible.

Marijuana plants go through a lot during their lifetime. There are going to be some major milestones, and when you become familiar with these, you will be able to take care of your plants better. You will be able to see any health problems if they come up before it harms the plant.

Once you know the best-case scenario, you will be able to see the problem and fix it immediately. But there might be times when you hit a problem that you just won't be able to fix.

You might have a plant that won't grow no matter what you do, but knowing exactly what to expect won't hurt. You will be able to see how much of a difference a couple of weeks will make. Once you are prepared for all stages of the plant's lifecycle by learning about all its behaviors and needs, you will have an abundant crop.

Seeds

As with most other plants, it all begins with a seed. Choose a seed and hold it in your hand. Turn it around. Look it over. Notice how heavy or light it is. See its color and shape.

Now, can you tell if that little seed will grow a female or male marijuana plant? You can't because nobody can. This introduces you to the main problem when trying to grow marijuana: is there any way that you can be certain that the seed you plant will produce the amount of marijuana you want?

This question is important since the female plant is the only one that produces the buds that you harvest to be smoked, vaped, dabbed, or ingested. The male plant doesn't produce any of this. A male plant could hurt your harvest if they are grown with female plants.

A male plant's main purpose is just to pollinate all the female plants. Even though this doesn't sound so bad, it can be. Once the female plant gets pollinated, it begins to use all its energy to produce the seeds. It stops using its energy to feed the buds that we want.

When you allow a male plant to grow beside female plants, this could cause a reduced bud harvest. It can also ruin all the euphoric properties that the female plant gives. Make sure you separate the female and male plants as quickly as possible.

It would be great to know if your seeds are going to make a female or male plant before you start growing them. Most seeds look alike, so the only way to know if the seed you are holding will be a female or male is to label it when you take it off the plant.

You can't label the seed, but you can put them in a container with seeds that are of the same sex. You don't need to store every single seed in its own container. You can fill a container with seeds as long as they are of the same sex and strain.

Any container will work. The only containers that won't work are plastic bags or any airtight container. Any moisture that gets trapped can cause the seed to mold, and then they are useless.

Whatever you put them in, make sure you mark it with the sex and strain so you can keep them separated.

Since cannabis uses sexual reproduction to make and spread seeds, one seed will get produced by two parents, and they will contain some genes from both female and male plants.

Underneath the seed's waxy coat, lies a small dehydrated plant just waiting to get exposed to warmth and moisture. The seed slows down its metabolism and enters a state of suspended animation. This keeps the seeds viable for a long time and possibly indefinitely.

When the seed receives heat and water, it will sprout. If not, it will get old and die. This is why you aren't able to keep seeds for a long time. Some seeds will keep longer and better than others.

Besides that tiny little plant in the seed is some calories that will help the plant start its journey. This is called the endosperm.

Seeds can stay dormant until they get exposed to light and water. Seeds are hardy and can survive well in cool, dark places as long as they have a stable temperature like in a cellar or fridge.

You have to protect your seeds because they can die. This means that they won't ever grow into a plant. You can stop this from happening by carefully storing them because extreme temperatures are the easiest way to damage the seeds. Temperatures that hit below freezing could kill the seeds.

Seeds and Moisture

I touched on this a bit above, but it needs to be emphasized more...

Moisture levels have to be kept as low as possible when you store your seeds. Fungus loves moisture, and this harms the seed. Moisture could also cause the seeds to sprout too early. Either one of these problems can interfere with growing plants that can be harvested.

Once you are ready to sprout your seeds, you are going to need moisture, but you still have to be careful that the seeds don't absorb too much moisture, or the seed might rot or mold.

Once you begin sprouting marijuana seeds, the moisture enters the seed through tiny openings called micropyles. If these get clogged or misshapen, it might be hard for them to germinate.

Seedlings

During this stage, there will be two embryonic leaves that will open from the stem. It does this to receive sunlight that it needs to get out of its seed casing. These leaves aren't going to look anything like an actual marijuana leaf that you are used to seeing.

The second set of leaves that grow will have the rounded points that make it stand out in a class all its own. This leaf is so recognizable that most people within the cannabis community use it to show their lifestyle.

The roots are also growing while the leave starts to grow and spread out from the plant's top. Very soon, new leaves are going to grow, and the plant will go into its first growth cycle. From this point, the plant will continue to grow until the buds begin to flower.

The seedling phase could last between one and three weeks, depending on:

- Light quality
- Light duration
- Humidity

- Airflow

- How much water the seed gets

- Marijuana strain being grown

- Type of soil

The only thing you need to focus on is growing a healthy plant instead of the time it is taking to get through all the stages. Don't worry about it if your seedlings are taking a bit longer to get through this phase. It is a plant, and it knows what it is doing.

As the plant starts developing its roots and foliage, it is going to transition into the vegetative stage. This is important if you are going to transplant your seedlings. This is the time to do it.

Vegetative Stage

This is the time when your cannabis plant starts growing those big jagged leaves that you have been waiting for. Your plant will produce more foliage since it will be able to absorb and process more nutrients and carbon dioxide.

During this growth stage, the roots are going to keep expanding, and the plant grows taller. You will be able to see your plant grow. A plant that is healthy could grow two inches in one day. The plant will grow from about eight inches into a two to three-foot-tall plant in about six weeks.

How long this phase lasts depends on the light it is exposed to. If you are growing the plants outside, it is going to depend on where you live. If you are growing inside, you can keep the plant in this stage for as long as you want. This stage normally takes one to two months.

There are a lot of things happening at this stage. To start with, the plant is growing stalks and leaves. It is producing a solid structure capable of supporting heavy buds. As the plant gets taller, new layers of leaves are growing, too. During this time, you will be able to see the differences between the strains of cannabis.

You should keep the temperature between 68 and 77 degrees with humidity content of about 50 to 70 percent. The plants need to have about 18 hours of white light daily and fertilizer when needed. This stage will last about one to two months.

You don't have to do much during this stage, but you need to pay attention to the light exposure. The cannabis plant will stop growing upwards when it begins getting less light each day. This is when the plant goes into the pre-flowering phase.

Flowering Stage

This is the last stage for the cannabis plant, and it is the most important. This stage starts after the plant isn't getting exposed to as much light. This is when the plant becomes sexually mature and is ready to spread some genes. Both the male and female plants have a flowering stage but the male plants normally mature earlier than females usually by a few weeks.

Once the plants reach this stage, they start producing huge amounts of sticky resin on its leaves. This resin contains the largest amounts of THC. This is the ingredient that you are after.

How potent the THC is gets determined by the time the plant gets to flower. It also depends on whether the plant got fertilized and pollinated.

You need to keep the male plants separated from the female plants. If the female plants get pollinated, it can ruin the amount of THC the plant produces. The females aren't going to produce seeds either if they don't get pollinated.

When you keep the female plants away from the male plants, it will produce sinsemilla. This basically means a female plant that won't have any seeds. These plants will produce huge amounts of resin and fake seedpods. Both of these will have huge amounts of THC, and this is what you are after.

Remember that you might have a hermaphroditic plant. This means your plant will have both sets of reproductive organs. These plants are able to pollinate themselves, and this can ruin your harvest. You have to find and destroy any hermaphroditic plants.

This flowering stage can last anywhere between six to ten weeks, but it could go on a bit longer. You can split up this stage into a few sections. This phase could happen right after your plant gets through its vegetative stage. You might notice your plants are developing some buds.

You are probably eager to harvest those buds you see, but you need to wait, and it might take some time. How long this takes depends on the strain you are growing and the amount of control you have on the growing environment.

Once the bud starts developing, the plant is flowering, and it has stopped growing because it is now investing everything into growing the buds. During this stage, your plants are going to need phosphorus and potassium based nutrients. These buds are covered in resin, heavy, and you will be able to smell them. Some of the pistils are going to turn brown, and some of the larger leaves on the bottom will turn yellow. These buds will produce milky white, thin, long pistils or hairs that will start emerging in the next eight to ten weeks.

Try to keep the temperature around 68 to 77 degrees with about 50 percent humidity. The plant still needs about 12 hours of light daily. If you fertilize regularly, you need to stop doing this about ten days before the plant is completely mature. You will know the plant is mature when the buds are smelly, glimmering, and dense.

Up until this point, the entire plant was green. During this time, the pistils are going to turn brown, the big leaves are going to turn yellow, and the buds are going to get heavier and expand. Depending on the strain of cannabis and the taste you are going after, you can start harvesting.

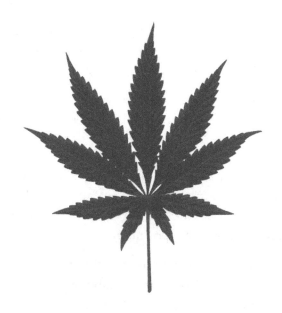

CHAPTER 2

CANNABIS STRAINS

◆◇◆

When you browse through different cannabis strains or you are exploring cannabis in a shop, you will likely notice that strains are broke up into three different groups: Sativa, Indica, and hybrid. Most consumers will use these types f cannabis as a touchstone for how they may affect you.

- It is believed that Indica strains are sedating, and are perfect for relaxing with a movie or to use as a nightcap before bed.

13

- Sativas provide an uplifting, invigorating cerebral effect that mixes well with creative projects, physical activity, and social gatherings.

- Hybrid fall somewhere between these two, and provide you with a balance between the effects of Indica and Sativa.

This belief of the different effects of sativas, indicas, and hybrids are so deeply rooted in our cannabis culture that budtenders will most often start their recommendations by asking you which type you prefer

But if you actually took a look at the chemical makeup of indicas and sativas, there cannabinoids and terpenes, you will see that there isn't a clear reason as to why one type would be uplifting and the other sedating. Indica and Sativa strains look very different, and they grow in a different manner, but this distinction is only really helpful for the grower.

We are going to look at the physical differences, but we're also going to look at why they may create a different type of high.

A Sativa plant is tall in stature and has narrow leaves. They have a longer flowering cycle, and they grow better in warm climates that have a long season. An Indica plant is shorter in stature, and their leaves are broader and connected. They have a shorter flowering cycle. They also do well in colder climates that have a shorter growing season.

What the Research Says

In order to find a strain that provides you with your de-sired effects, your best bet is to try and learn the chemi-cal makeup of the strain. It is definitely efficient for the first-timer to use the Sativa, Indica, and hybrid systems. With the sheer amount of strains out there, where else could we start?

The problem is, the Indica and Sativa system is non-sense. How a plant grows does not play a part in what kind of effects it will have on a person when ingested. There is no scientific or factual basis for making sweep-ing recommendations based on the type of plants. This means that just because it is a Sativa, does not mean it is going to energize. Just like not all indicas will sedate you.

But, if you want to know for certain how a strain will make you feel, you will want to learn about terpenes and cannabinoids. Also, the effects that any given strain will have on you will depend on several factors, which include their chemical makeup, your biology and toler-ance, consumption method, and dose.

Let's look at cannabinoids. Cannabinoids lead the pack of chemicals that create the effects of cannabis. The two most common ones are THC and CBD. THC is what makes you feel high and hunger, and relieves the symp-toms of nausea, pain, and more. CBD is non-intoxicat-ing and can help alleviate inflammation, pain, anxiety, and other ailments.

There are other cannabinoids in cannabis, but THC and CBD should be the ones you should worry about learning right now. When making a selection on what strain you want, consider their THC and CBD contents instead of whether it is Indica or Sativa.

A THC dominant stain is going to provide you with the most euphoric experience. These are also the plants that are normally picked by those treating insomnia, anxiety, depression, pain, and more. If THC heavy strains make you feel anxious or don't like the side effects associated with it, you can choose strains that are higher in CBD.

A CBD dominant strain has only a small amount of THC and is used by people who are sensitive to THC or people who need to remain clear-headed.

A balanced THC and CBD strain will have levels of THC and CBD that are similar, which provides a mild euphoria with symptom relief. These are often a good choice for first-time consumers looking for an introduction into a cannabis high.

Both Indica and Sativa strains can have different cannabinoid profiles.

Terpenes are the other part of the chemical makeup of cannabis that plays a part in how it affects you. If you have ever used aromatherapy to help invigorate or relax your body and mind, you already have a basic understanding of terpenes. They are the aromatic compounds produced by fruit and plants. They are secreted by the same glands that release CBD and THC, and terpenes are what makes cannabis smell like pine, berries, fuel, citrus, and so on.

Various types of terpenes are found in cannabis, and it is worth learning about the most common ones, especially terpinolene, limonene, caryophyllene, and myrcene because they are the ones the most likely to occur in high levels. You'll want to study the seeds you are considering to purchase and find one that will have an aroma that you will want. If you have a local dispensary, you can always go in and see if you can smell some of their buds to pick out the one you like the smell of.

Lastly, you should think about the following questions when it comes to picking out your best strain.

1. How much experience with cannabis do you have? If you have a low tolerance, think about going with a low THC strain.

2. Are you prone to anxiety or other THC side effects? If you are, then you should go with a high CBD strain.

Answering these questions can help you to figure out what strains of cannabis you should consider growing. After all, you want to grow cannabis that you are going to want to use.

With that in mind, we are going to look at 12 different strains and how they can affect you. Remember, though; there are many, many more cannabis strains out there if none of these tickle your fancy.

Most Common Cannabis Strains

Different types of cannabis are going to interact with your body's receptors in different ways. This means that the mental and physical effects they cause will vary. There are a couple of different factors that go into determining the type of experience you may experience, which we have already covered. So, here are some of the more common cannabis strains you may come across.

- Skunk No. 1

This is a hybrid strain that has had a global influence in the cannabis world, and it has parented a horde of Skunk crosses since it was first grown in the 1970s. As you could guess by the name, it radiates with an aromatic blend of subtle earthy notes and sour skunkiness. This hybrid can provide you with creativity through its high energy buzz as appetite loss and stress melt away. It has a 29.2% active THC testing rate.

- Strawberry Guava

According to its name, this strain has a fruity flavor profile, which provides you with a well-rounded hybrid experience. Strawberry guava will offer you the best of both worlds by finding the perfect balance between that cerebral feeling and a mellowed-out euphoria. This is great for anxiety relief and relaxation.

- Green Crack

Green crack provides you with and herbal and peppery flavor profile. There are very few strains that compare to the sharp focus and energy of green crack. It provides you with an invigorating mental buzz that will keep you going. It also has a tangy and fruity flavor similar to a mango and is a great daytime strain that can help fight depression, fatigue, and stress.

- Papaya Punch

This strain brings a punch of fruity flavor. It is a fresh flavored Indica. It has tropical berry notes and relaxing vibes. This is a great choice if you are looking to knock out at the end of a long day or if you simply want to relax with your favorite book. Papaya punch is a great strain to help you chill out.

- Bruce Banner

Bruce Banner is more well known as his alter-ego The Incredible Hulk, but he probably wouldn't be so stressed out by all of his anger if he has some of his namesakes. This strain also has some hidden strength due to its very high THC content. It is powerful, and its effects hit quickly and are strong. It sometimes settles into a creative and euphoric buzz. The effects tend to be heavy in the head, but it can bring about some relaxation to the body, which makes it a good daytime bud.

- Bubble Gum

Bubble gum has a long history that has taken it all across the world before they finally produced a stable bubble gum that has its characteristic euphoric high and sweet smell.

- White Widow

White widow is one of the most famous strains around the world. It is a balanced hybrid. It has been a part of every Dutch coffee shop since it came about in the 1990s. Its buds are white and contain a crystal resin, which lets you know it has a potent effect. A powerful burst of energy and euphoria breakthrough immediately and will stimulate your creativity and conversation. White widow flowers in around 60 days indoors.

- Sunset Sherbet

This is an Indica-leaning hybrid that has intoxicatingly potent effects. It holds the genetic lineage of its GSC parent. Sherbet has some powerful full-body effects which are increased by its jolt of cerebral energy. It has a very complex aroma with notes of candy, sweet berry, and skunky citrus. Sour moods, stress, and tension will melt away into a carefree mindset and relaxation.

- Blueberry

Blueberry won the Cannabis Cup in 2000 as Best Indica. Its history dates back to the late 1970s. It contains sweet flavors of blueberries and has some relaxing effects to help provide you with a long-lasting euphoria. A lot of consumers will use blueberry to help with stress and pain.

- AK-47

Despite its powerful name, AK-47 helps to leave you mellow and relaxed. It is a Sativa-dominant strain and has a complex blend of effects and flavors. It can provide you with a steady and long-lasting heady buzz that helps to keep you engaged and alert in social or creative activities.

- Bubba Kush

Bubba kush is an Indica strain and is known for its tranquilizing effects. It has subtle notes of coffee and chocolate and delights the palate as its relaxing effects take over. From top to bottom, muscles will relax with heaviness as the dreamy euphoria blankets you and gets rid of stress and bringing about happy moods.

- Sour Diesel

Sour Diesel is an invigorating Sativa-dominant strain that gets its name due to its pungent, diesel-like aroma. It is a fast-acting strain that will provide you with an energizing and dreamy cerebral effect. Depression, stress, and pain will fade away with long-lasting relief from sour diesel.

Now with all of that in mind, you can start to think about what strain, or strains, you would like to grow.

CHAPTER 3

PREPARING YOUR SEEDS

— ◆ ◇ ◆ —

Germination is when a new plant starts growing from seeds. This is sometimes called "popping." This is the first step when beginning your cannabis plants. You can get cannabis seeds from many different sources, and these can vary in quality.

When you are getting your seeds, you need to make sure they are mature, and they are dark brown with light accents and they feel hard. You don't want seeds that look green and feel fresh. This shows that the seed hasn't matured.

After you have bought your cannabis seeds, be sure you have enough space to let your plants grow to be big and healthy. Don't plant seeds if you aren't sure of your intentions, available time, and grow space.

Ways to Germinate

Cannabis seeds are just like any other seed. They need three things to be able to germinate: air, heat, and water. Due to this, there are several ways to germinate your seeds. The simplest and most common way involves paper towels that have been saturated with water.

- Paper Towel Method

You are going to need seeds, paper towels, two clean plates, and of course, water.

Take four paper towels and soak them with water. They need to be wet but not have water running out of them.

Take two of the wet paper towels and place them on a plate. Put the cannabis seeds one inch apart and cover them with the other two paper towels.

To make a protected, dark place, put another plate on top of the seeds. Place it so that the plates create a dome effect.

Put them in a place where they will be warm. The perfect temperature would be between 70 and 90 degrees.

Once you have done all of this, now you get to wait. You can check on the paper towels from time to time to make sure they are still wet. If they feel a bit dry, mist them with a bit more water to keep them happy.

You might notice that some of the seeds seem to germinate faster than others. You will know that a seed has germinated when the seed pops open, and a sprout appears.

This will be your taproot and will turn into the stem of your plant. You have just had a successful germination. You have to keep this area clean and sterile. Don't touch the seeds or taproot when it starts splitting.

- Soaking the Seeds

This is another good method to help your seeds germinate. Place your seeds in a glass of room temperature water overnight. This will trigger a hormone that tells the cells to begin germinating.

Make sure you don't leave the seeds in water longer because this could cause the seeds to be oxygen-deprived, they might drown, and this causes them to rot.

Once you let the seeds soak, take them out of the water and put them on one of these:

- Light soilless mixture
- Cheesecloth
- Any growing medium
- Moist paper towels

Put the seeds in a warm place and make sure whatever you put them on stays moist.

If you accidentally get the growing medium too wet, make sure you drain off as much water as possible to keep the seed from drowning. If you used a cheesecloth or paper towel, in a few days, you will start to see a sprout coming out of the seed.

If you used growing mediums for germination, you are going to have to wait. Make sure you don't open the growing medium or dig around in the dirt. If you do, you are running the risk of injuring the seed.

If you see fungus developing while the seeds are germinating, you can mist it with a very mild fungicide or bleach solution. Be careful that you don't damage or kill your seed.

When the seed has developed a white sprout, you can carefully pick it up and plant it. Make sure you have a growing medium handy that you can plant it in. The tiny rootlet is extremely sensitive, and too much light or air can damage it. If you plant the seedling cover it with just a sprinkling of dirt. Make sure the white tip is pointing down.

CHAPTER 4

GERMINATION AND PLANTING

———————— ◆◇◆ ————————

Like with any type of gardening, cannabis growing is a skill that you are going to have to develop. It is fairly easy to learn, but it will take a lifetime for you to master. You should not be intimated by growing your own plant. It is not all that complicated, and you can make it as expensive or inexpensive as you want.

Once you are ready to start planting, the first thing you are going to have to do is make sure you have a good location set up. You have the option to grow your plants inside or outside. Having an indoor setup will give you complete control over the growing process, like how much light they get. However, indoor growing also comes with a number of responsibilities because the cannabis plant will depend on you to survive.

If you choose to grow your plants outside, it will be less expensive because nature will do the biggest part of the work, like providing your plants with light. However, outdoor growing sites tend to not be as private as people would want them to be, and growers will often have to deal with their plants getting stolen or messed up by local animals. You will have to weigh these options in order to figure out which one is going to work best for you.

Once you have that figured out, you will move onto deciding on your growing medium. Your plant is going to need a medium that will provide it with the needed nutrients in order to develop the perfect buds. There are many different options when it comes to growing mediums. Every medium comes with its own requirements, like how often it will need to be watered, but at the end of the day, each option is equally capable of growing a healthy cannabis plant.

The most common and the easiest to use option would be soil. Ideally, you will want to use well-composted organic soil that is full of nutrients that will help the cannabis grow. If you aren't using a soil that has been optimized for growing cannabis, you will want to make sure that it contains perlite to make sure that it drains well.

There is also the option to go soilless. You could use coco coir, vermiculite, or other soilless mixtures. While these can become more expensive, they do come with a few advantages, like reducing the chance of having to deal with pests and diseases that live in the soil. They also have disadvantages. The main one is that they don't contain nutrients for the plant, so you are going to have to provide your plants with the proper nutrient in the right amounts at the right time.

Lastly, you could choose to grow them in a hydroponic garden. This is where you grow them directly in water.

This method can help you to produce very high yields, but there is a pretty steep learning curve, and it also ends up getting very expensive.

Along the same lines, you will want to make sure that you select the right nutrients. Cannabis is easy to grow, but nutrients are able to improve your end results. When it comes to marijuana, you are going to want to use specific nutrients that are going to help your plant thrive during its various growth stages. Those nutrients will need to be formulated for the medium you have chosen to use. Certain nutrients will only work in a hydroponic system, while others work better in soil.

You will also need to think about the pH levels of your water. If you use the incorrect pH, the nutrients aren't going to be able to be absorbed by the plants. The medium will also have to be considered when it comes to figuring out the right pH.

You will also have to make sure that your cannabis is kept at the appropriate temperature. Cannabis is hardy and can survive well in heat and cold. But just like us, it will get stressed and not work properly in extremes. Your cannabis seeds can boil or freeze to death. Growth will stop. It can hit survival mode if the temperatures go to one extreme or another for too long. 80.6 degrees is the ideal temperature for vigorous growth. This is easy to achieve indoors using fans, AC units, and cooling and heating mats.

If you are growing outside, you are going to have to pick the right time. You will need to know your climate well. Having a sun cycle app or a chart can help you to get your timing right. Planting them too early, and you will run the risk of your plants going into flower immediately, then re-vegging once daylight increases. This is not what you want. The flowers aren't going to form properly when the blooming starts. If you wait too late, you will end up having small plants with fewer flowers.

Now is the time when you can use that well-prepared seed. Place those seeds into a ½ inch hold in a small pot using seedling soil. This soil does not need to have as many nutrients to start with. It is best to use a soil that is made for seedlings and has low quantities of nutrients. Plants are susceptible to nutrient burn during this time if they get too many nutrients.

Each seed should be given its own pot. Place the seed into the hole and then cover it with the soil. Spray the soil with water. This will tamp it down, so you don't need to press on the soil. The seed will continue to germinate over the next week, and the plant should begin to surface at that point. The taproot will make other root offshoots to keep the plant-strong.

During this time, you should use a plant sprayer to keep the soil moistened. Water is very important at this early stage. Plants who don't get enough water will compensate by not growing up to the fullest capacity. Too much water can cause the plant to miss out on needed oxygen. Leaves will begin to wither, and then the plant and growing medium will become more susceptible to bacteria and disease.

The soil needs to be kept adequately moist. It won't need a lot of water, but water evaporates fast. This is why you should not place seedlings next to windowsills or heaters. Mist them one to two times during the day.

During this time, you will want to make sure that you keep your plant exposed to adequate light through a grow light. We will talk about different grow lights in a later chapter.

As soon as you see the seedlings pop their heads out of the soil, it is important that you inspect to see how far the plant is from the light. Make sure that heat from the light hitting the plant never goes past 72 degrees. You should consider to mist them about two times a day.

After its first two internodes appear, you can start feeding it with some root-stimulating foliar nutrients. You should start with small doses as the roots can stand higher concentrations yet. They will grow about half an inch each day. If the leaf tips start looking burned, you are giving them too many nutrients.

Once the roots start growing out of the bottom, you will then transplant them into a bigger pot. Otherwise, the plant will become root-bound and stop growing. Now the biggest part of the growth takes place.

CHAPTER 5

VEGETATIVE GROWTH

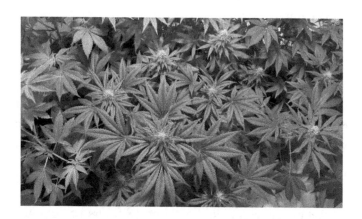

Every plant will have some similarities in the way they grow, but the cannabis plant has some quirks that set them apart from others. There are some steps that you do during the vegetative stage that will benefit you later in the plant's life like what to feed the plant and when you need to feed it.

During this stage, the plant will focus on getting strong and larger. When any plant is just growing leaves and stems without buds, the plant is in the vegetative stage.

If you are growing your cannabis inside, you can keep your plants in this stage for as long as you would like by giving them 18 hours of light each day. This can be accomplished by using a timer and grow lights.

Outdoor growers who rely on the sun to get the plants to the point of making buds, don't have as much control over their plants as indoor growers do. Indoor growers can control the final shape and size of their plants.

There is an exception to this rule, and that is auto-flowering cannabis strains. These varieties will go from start to harvest in three months no matter the amount of light they get.

When you expose them to light for about 18 hours daily will make cannabis think that it is growing time. As long as they get this amount of light, they will stay in this vegetative stage. They will only grow leaves and stems.

People who grow their cannabis indoors normally give them an 18 – 6 or 24 – 0 schedule during this stage. The 18 – 6 means you give the plants 18 hours of light and six hours of darkness every day. The 24 – 0 schedule means you are giving the plant 24 hours of light without any darkness.

Some growers say the 24 – 0 is best while others say the 18 – 6 is best, so which one is actually better?

Well, your answer will depend on who you ask. It could also be different for various strains, too. Most strains are fine and will do great when they are given 24 hours of light daily. Other strains do better on the 18 – 6.

If the cost of electricity is a major concern, you might want to think about doing the 18 – 6 schedule to help keep your electricity costs down. This lets you use the six hours of darkness to cool the area. If the growing area gets too hot, you could set the six hours of darkness to be during this time. This basically means that the lights won't be burning during the hottest part of the day.

If you worry about the temperature getting below 70 degrees, then the 24 hours of light would be a better choice since it keeps your plants warm.

There are going to be growers who thing their plants need a dark time to have the best growth, but others think that more light hours are better because they give your plants faster growth during the vegetative stage.

Auto-flowering marijuana strains will need the 18 – 6 schedule from seed to harvest. You treat them like they are in the vegetative stage and just let them do what they do best.

An 18 – 6 schedule is normal for all plants during their vegetative stage. It is simple, easy, and the plants grow healthy and fast. If you live in hotter climates and worry about high electricity costs, the six hours without lights is very helpful.

I have done the 24, 22, and 20 hours of lights daily, and they grew fine. If you have figured out your perfect number, the biggest difference is that the plants will just grow faster. A complete day of light will give you faster growth since the plants get more light to create energy. It is completely up to you to figure out which schedule is best for you. Basically, anything that is between 18 and 24 hours each day will be fine.

Most growers who grow indoors will let their plants vegetate between four and eight weeks. Seedling could begin to flower three weeks from the time they germinated, but the plants are going to be a lot smaller. Most growers will let their plants vegetate longer since you are giving them more growing time to get bigger plants. This will also give you larger yields if you have enough light to cover all the plants. With that said, you will still be producing a lot of buds with many plants growing at one time if you fill up your grow space.

During this growth period, the plant will build its root system and stems. After it has created good stems and roots, will it begin to grow foliage. During this time, your plant needs lots of nitrogen.

The early leaves start the photosynthesis process by absorbing the sun and helping the plant grow more. Once the plants have germinated and started to stabilize, think about getting rid of any seeds that haven't germinated or any seedling that is growing. By doing this, they won't be competing with the other plants for nutrients and light.

When the plant has established a stable root system, and you have your environment set up the right way, you will just need some upkeep to get a good harvest. Your plants will continue to develop and grow if you give them the right amount of light and nutrients. They will develop a strong structure that is needed for the flowering stage.

While your plants are continuing to mature and develop, they are going to need more light, water, fertilizer, and more carbon dioxide. They are also going to need more nitrogen. You need to make sure you are giving the plant all it needs.

First Leaves

The leaves of the cannabis plant grow in phases. Every phase can produce a specific number of leaves. The first phase will produce one leaf. The next phase will grow three leaves. The third phase will make five leaves, etc.

The amount of leaves that get produced in one phase normally stops at about ten. You might see some leaves called "lamina" in some literature.

After a couple of weeks of growth, your plants will have experienced about six various rounds of growth. They should be producing a steady and regular amount of leaves with each new phase. You might see that they are developing and expanding branches outward.

Feeding Your Seedlings

You need to make sure that your young plants get a lot of nitrogen early during their development. You can use fertilizers that are made from bat guano, blood meal, or worm meal. They will help you get all the nutrients your plants are going to need from organic sources.

There are other options that include fish compounds, nettle blends, or algae compounds. There are many factors that make fertilizers that are organic the best choice. The main reason is that it is better and you could overfeed your plants. This might damage them when you are using chemical fertilizers.

Once the first leaves pop out, you are going to want to measure how much electrical conductance the nutrient solution has. It needs to be as close to one as possible. When the plant begins to grow and mature, it is fine for the electrical conductance to go higher. Once the plant has about five levels of foliage, you can raise the electrical conductance again to around 1.5.

When you have branches on your plants, you can bring the electrical conductance to two, but be careful about the amount of nutrient solution and water. If you over water your plants, it could cause them to grow more stem than buds. This is counterproductive for many growers.

Let your plant's root systems air out and rest between irrigation times. Add lots of nitrogen to the plants when they first develop leaves, just make sure you keep the electrical conductance at about one.

Environmental Factors

The environment that your plants are growing in needs to optimized along every stage of growth but especially during the early stages. You have a few options with lighting.

Once your plants are past the seedling phase, you can give them light for an entire day, but is it best to stimulate night to give the plants some darkness. You need metal halide or sodium vapor lamps to be sure you are giving them the correct type of light.

You need to keep the temperature somewhere between 68 and 78 degrees. The roots can be a bit cooler at about 65 degrees. Despite all this, be sure the soil is warm, especially in the early stages. It the roots don't grow properly, the entire plant won't either.

Don't forget about the humidity in the room, too. This is going to affect how well your plant breathes and how healthy the plant is. You need the humidity in the room to be between 50 and 70 percent. Once the plant reaches maturity, it won't be as sensitive to humidity.

Controlling these factors are going to help optimize your plant. Remember that genetics still plays a large role in figuring out how the plant is going to develop and what kind of yield you will get. Even though you have everything perfect, you won't be able to turn bad genetics into great products. If you are careful and meticulous during the cultivation process, you can still optimize the plant no matter how high its yield might be.

Daily Care

While your plants are in the vegetative phase, your job is fairly simple. Your plants will grow fast, and they are fairly tough during this stage. In order to keep your plants healthy and happy, you are going to do the following:

- Air Circulation

Your cannabis plants need to have a constant supply of fresh air, so your plants get the carbon dioxide they need to grow. Keep the air moving so you don't have any hot spots and the leaves are constantly moving. If you are growing the plants outside, you might want to put up windbreaks if it were to get too windy so your plants don't get blown around too violently.

- Not Too Hot or Cold

Plants in the vegetative phase, like having a comfortable room temperature or a bit warmer. Stay away from low humidity in this stage if at all possible. Don't expose your plants to freezing temperatures.

- Give Them Light

If you have grow lights, use them as directed. Just turn them on and keep it off of your plants. Normally they are placed a couple of inches above the plants. Outdoor plants will vegetate until the days begin getting shorter. Indoor plants can stay in the vegetative phase as long as you want them to, and you are giving them at least 18 hours of light.

- Nutrients

If you are giving your plants nutrients, begin using a nu-trient schedule at half the strength. Only raise the nutri-

ent levels if they are needed. Just add the number of nutrients needed to your water before you give it to your
plants or add it to a reservoir. You will need to manage
the pH levels if you use liquid nutrients.

- Give Them Water

Seedlings won't need as much water until they start
growing very fast. Especially if your young plants are in
larger containers. Don't give them a lot of water until
the plants are growing well. When the plant is growing
new stems and leaves regularly, begin watering them
this way:

- Adding nutrients to the water

o Wait until the top of the growing medium is dry.
Stick your finger in the soil to see if it is dry.

o Add water until you see about 20 percent runoff
draining out of the pot.

o Do step one again

o If it takes a long time for the water to come out
of the bottom, or if the pot takes longer than five
days to dry out, you might have a drainage problem.

- Growing without nutrients

o Give them just enough water that the growing
medium is moistened but not enough to get run-

o   Don't accidentally wash away the extra nutrients because you aren't giving them any more

o   Watch out for overwatering. Soil that is rich enough to give your plants the nutrients it needs until it is ready to be harvested could easily be overwatered.

Some growers will lift the pot to figure out if you need to water the plants. You get to decide which way is easiest for you.

You need to water your plants when the top inch of soil feels dry. If your plants are in containers, you need to be sure that the water can drain easily out of the bottom. If you have a hydroponic setup, they will always have lots of water.

This growth period will be followed by the flowering stage. It is your job to give your plants what they need to grow properly before they begin to flower.

This means they need to have healthy foliage and a tough structure so they can hold up the weight of the buds. They also need a strong, healthy root system. Watch the temperature, carbon dioxide, nutrients, and light in your grow room during this process.

This is especially important during this phase. You need to be careful when you are watering and irrigating your plants. As the plants get larger, they will need more water to keep up with their development.

This basically means that it will be easy for the plant to get dehydrated during this time. Be on the lookout for yellowing or curling leaves and monitor your nutrient solution if you are using a hydroponics system.

Nutrients, Humidity, and Temperature

When your plants get to their peak growth phase, you can begin exposing your plants to an entire day of light, if you want to. In my experience, it is best to do the 18 – 6 schedule. Using metal halide or sodium vapor lights will give you the perfect light.

Remember to keep the temperature in the room around 68 and 78 degrees. The roots can be kept at a slightly lower temperature. Just make sure the soil is warm enough, especially when they are in the early stages of growth. The roots need to develop in order for the rest of the plant to develop correctly.

Make sure you check the temperature where your plants experience the most heat and that is right under the light. If you can't hold your hand under the light for longer than ten seconds, it is too hot for your plants, and you need to bring the temperature down. If it is just a hot spot, you can use fans to move the heat and give better air circulation.

Cannabis can't handle cold temperatures. If the temperature hits freezing, it can kill your plants. If you keep your plants in a cooler area like your basement, take any steps you need to in order to make sure the bottoms of the plants have a protective barrier from the cold.

Remember to monitor the humidity in the room, too. This effects how well your plants breathe. You need the humidity in the room to be between 50 and 70 percent. Once the plant matures, it won't be as sensitive to humidity.

You will need to continue to add nitrogen. You need the electrical conductance to be between 1.5 and 2. If you use soil, be sure you are adding liquid fertilizers and monitor the soil's moisture.

What About Problems

You have to keep a close watch on your plants during the first few times you grow cannabis. You will make a mistake because everybody does. Good growers will always watch their plants closely so they can catch and fix any problems before the plant gets damaged permanently.

It is fine to make a mistake, just watch for them and fix them. Cannabis plants are fairly resilient, especially during the vegetative phase. As long as you correct the problem that is bothering them, they normally bounce back and will produce buds. Nutrient deficiencies and problems during the vegetative phase won't have much effect on the flowering stage if the problems are fixed quickly.

Be on the lookout for:

- Look for signs of bugs like spots, eggs, mucus trails, etc.

- Look for "stretching" or when your plant grows taller with a lot of space between leaves rather than growing a lot of leaves and getting bushy. This means that your plant needs more light and is trying to find the sun.

- Slow growth meant there is something wrong.

- Watch out for mold on leaves or buds. If you see things on your buds or leaves that don't look like resin, you might be seeing mold. Mold looks like white powder on the leaves.

- If you smell something bad coming from your plants, it usually indicated rotting, mold, or bacteria. Look at your system and find the bad smell. If they begin smelly skunky, this is perfectly normal.

- Watch for leaves falling off, dying, or curling fairly fast. If your plant loses more leaves that it is growing, you have a problem.

- Strange spots or coloring on the leaves. It is normal for the lower leaves to turn brown or yellow and die while the plant is maturing. It is also normal for the leaves to begin turning yellow in the last week or so before it is time to harvest as the plant is pulling nitrogen from the leaves to take it to the mature buds. Other than these exceptions, your leaves need to look healthy and green.

Don't start worrying about everything. If you feel like your plant is having a problem, see if you can find out what it is and try to fix it as quickly as possible. Most of the time these problems can be fixed if they are found during the early growth stages.

How Long is the Vegetative Stage

This gets determined by you. Most cannabis plants will need no less than three weeks in this stage before they begin making flowers. Once that happens, you get to choose how long your plant stays in this phase. You are the only one who can "flip the switch" and allow your plants to move into the next phase of their lives. If your plants are auto-flowering, you don't have any control over this.

When you begin your plants from seed, even if it is an auto-flowering strain, you will always have between two and three weeks of vegetative growth before the buds begin forming, and it won't matter what you do. Most growers will let their plants stay in the vegetative phase from a couple of weeks to a couple of months.

How large your plant gets during this phase can affect your final yield because larger plants will produce more buds than smaller plants will. You will need enough light to cover all the buds, or they won't develop properly. Light is the food for buds to grow.

Figuring Out the Sex

There are two methods that are used to determine the gender of your cannabis plants. Gender is something that you absolutely need to know because mixing female and male plants can ruin your crop.

The first way to determine the gender is to look at the fifth series of leaves on the plant. You will want to do this just before the plant is supposed to flower. Hybrids with Indica genetics and indicas will show their sex between the leaves of the plant just before they flower.

When you look carefully, you should see a small white fiber if the plant is a female. A male plant will have a small ball rather than a tendril or fiber. This isn't easy to figure out, and it isn't the most reliable. It can be hard to find the sex organs of the plant since they are extremely small.

The easiest way is to do cuttings. When your plant is in a vegetative phase, take a cutting from the plant and then root them in a separate room. Expose the rooted cutting to 12 hours of light and dark. The plant should flower in a few days. If any are male, you will need to remove them from the growing room.

CHAPTER 6

CLONING

◆ ◇ ◆

While it may sound like a mad science experiment, you can clone your cannabis plant. Cloning gives you the ability to start growing another plant without having to start it from a seed and is a lot easier than you may think.

When it comes to reproducing cannabis, you have two options. You can either grow them from seed, where you will have to get a seed, germinate them, sex them out, and then continue the growing process. Seeds are formed through sexual reproductions, which you will need to cross a male and female plant through pollination to do. Then the females will produce more seeds. When you breed a male and female plant, you have the chance to create a hybrid of the parent plants.

Since sexual reproduction means that there is a random combination of the parents' characteristics, you won't know how it will taste or effect you until you use it. Just like with humans, every plant that is grown from seed will have a unique makeup due to genetics.

The second way is to create a plant is with cloning, which is called asexual reproduction. Simply put, a clone is a cutting that will always be identical to the plant it is taken off of.

By cloning, you will be able to make a brand new plant that will have the same makeup as the plants you like the most. Since it has identical genetics, a clone helps to provide you with a plant that has the same characteristics as the mother, like the grow time, yield, cannabinoid profile, flavor, and so on. If you were to come across a specific phenotype or strain you absolutely love, you may want to clone it in order to reproduce more buds with the same effects.

Cloning gives you a reliable way to make sure that your plants stay high quality. You will already know everything about how they act, grow, and taste. The genetic line won't change. There are some cannabis farmers that have been able to keep a cloned line going for nearly two decades. A single mother has the ability to produce over 50 clones each week.

Cloning is really the only guarantee, or close to it, that you will have in raising cannabis. After you have had a successful season, it is smart to clone one of your plants to improve your odds of having another successful season.

With cloning, you aren't going to have to get new seeds each time you want to grow another plant. All you have to do is take a cutting from the old one. You also won't have to deal with germinating the seed or sexing them out and getting rid of all the males. Not having to go through all of these steps is going to save you some time and space, and both of those is going to save you money.

For the outdoor grower, cloning works the best when they live an area with long growing seasons. Even with a really long growing season, you can't expect that those clones are going to get to their complete height since they often won't start growing until about three months into the growing season. That said, even clones that don't get a chance to grow large will have the ability to have amazing yields, and will develop a top full of buds.

The majority of people who clone plants will choose to take a bottom branch from the mother plant since these have naturally received less light, and are already struggling to survive. If you end up taking around two and four of the branches off of each of your plants you can, at least, double your total yield. While cloning tends to be risk-free because it doesn't pose a threat to the mother plant, clones will often die before they can root. It is very common for a person to take ten clones, and only one of them makes it to being planted, so make sure that you don't get discouraged if a lot of your clones end up dying and not producing a plant.

How to Clone

The cloning process is relatively easy and will require just a few items:

- Rooting hormone
- Rooting setup
- Razor
- Scissors

First, you will need to start out by choosing a setup and rooting medium. The most common mediums include rooting cubes, rockwool, or another non-soil equivalent such as foam or peat. Rockwool is simply a melted rock that has been spun to create a fine thread, and it is great at moisture retention and airflow. These cubes can be found in most grow stores.

If you are using these cubes, you are going to want to get a tray, a tray-cell insert, and a dome. The clone will be placed inside of the cubes, then that is placed in the tray-cells, and then that is set in the tray that has the water. To make sure that the humidity stays up, you should cover your tray with a dome, and you might want to use a heat mat.

Another way to do this is to use an auto-cloner. These will cut down on how much labor is going to be needed in order to feed and care for your clones. Using aeroponics, the setup will spray your cuttings with nutrient water at different times to get the roots to start growing. These tend to be more expensive than using the traditional root cube setup, but they are growing in popularity.

You will need to experiment to see which setup is going to work best for you. No matter what method you pick, make sure that your clones remain in a lot of light during the day, around 18 hours, and that there is plenty of humidity.

The Proper Way to Take a Cutting

The cloning process begins by picking out a mother plant. Make sure you aren't hasty in picking one out. When you are choosing a mother plant to make a clone from, look for plants that are the healthiest and study, and they should be at least two months into the vegetative cycle. You should not take a cutting from a plant that has begun to flower. If a cutting is taken from a flowering plant, it is a lot harder for it to take root, which increases its mortality rate. There is a small chance that it will root, but there will be differences.

You want to choose a plant that is hardy, has great yields, grows rapidly, has strong buds, and large roots. Outdoor and indoor-grown cannabis can be cloned, but you should always try to keep the clones in an environment that they are used to. Basically, outside plants should be cloned outside and vice versa. Don't try to bring an outside plant in.

If you are cloning your plants for the first time, you may not have a good understanding of your plants in order to know which one you should choose. Regardless, if you make sure you pick a female plant in the vegetative growth stage that seems healthy, then you are likely making a good choice, and it should work fine for cloning.

At a minimum, you need to go with a plant that is two months old or older. If you take a cutting before they reach two months, then they may not be mature enough to develop roots.

In order to take a cutting, stop fertilizing the mother plant for a couple of days before. This is going to allow nitrogen to work out of the leaves. When taking a cutting, excess nitrogen living in the leaves and stems will end up causing your clones to try and grow vegetation instead of using all of their energy to create roots.

It is also best to pick your clones from plants that were originally grown from regular seeds and not seeds that had been feminized. Cannabis plants that have been forced to produce feminized seeds are stressed to do so. If the plants created from those seeds are stressed out again, then they may end up becoming a hermaphrodite. You also shouldn't use a plant grown from auto-flowering seeds because they won't have enough time to grow before they start to flower, which will ruin your yields. Some people also find that that sativas tend to clone easier than indicas.

Make sure that you work in a sterile environment. Use disinfected scissors and razors and use gloves.

Look for a branch that is healthy and sturdy. You need to have at least two nodes on your final cutting, so make sure that you choose a branch that is long and healthy. A sturdy cutting is going to create a sturdy plant. You will want to make sure that you will end up with a six to eight-inch branch.

Cut your clone off of the mother right above the node on the mother plant. You can use scissors here. It could be hard for you to get a razor into the middle of the plant. The important thing is to make sure that whatever you use to cut with is very sharp. Make sure your instrument isn't dull because it will end up crushing the stem and will make forming the roots a lot harder.

Once you have your cutting, use a razor and cut right below the node on the bottom at a 45-degree angle. This will give it more surface area to help your plant start rooting from and will promote faster growth.

Immediately place your brand new cutting into some rooting hormone. Then place this into a rooting cube. If you have chosen to use an auto-cloner, you will place the rooting hormone into the cloner after you have taken your cuttings.

After you are don't taking a cutting, you should get rid of unnecessary leaves that are at the bottom and remove the tips from the rest of the leaves on your cutting. You will also want to make sure that you have at least one pair of leaves on your branch so that it will create two new branches. This will help to support its photosynthesis process, which will help your clones to take in water and nutrients.

Viral Infections Caused By Cloning

If you make sure that you pick out a healthy mother plant, your clones have a greater chance of being healthy as well. But there are times when a clone's characteristics can differ from its mother. For example, a clone group could end up having poor potassium uptake, which will end up causing the leaves to twist. This is not like their mother plant. This problem will become a bigger problem as more clones are formed.

When one of these plants are placed in a hydroponic system with plants from a different line, the second clone will start to show signs of poor potassium uptake. It is likely that a virus could have infected the first group, and then it got spread through the water into the other plants.

A mother plant has the ability to create thousands of clones during its lifetime. Unfortunately, the longer these clones are formed, the higher the chances are that they will develop a viral infection. Usually, annual plants have the ability to fight off these types of infections because the virus does not enter the seeds. This is why a germinated plant starts off free of infection, but can still face some challenges.

However, when a mother plant has been infected, the disease will be able to spread via the tissue, and you will be using that tissue to create your clones. There is a slight chance that a virus could end up being spread to plants through planting mediums, air, or water Much like humans, as plants age, they have a higher risk of being infected with something, which can cause the older mothers to be at a higher risk of infecting their clones.

Clones can end up ruining the natural anti-infection defense that cannabis has. Instead of only living for a few months like they are supposed to, the plant gets to live for many years by way of the clones. With time, the odds of those viral infections will grow. While the chance of infection gets larger over time, there is still a chance that you can have a garden full of healthy, potent clones that are several generations old. Most growers report that there aren't any noticeable changes.

Transplanting

You will want to check on your clones every day to make sure that they have plenty of water by check the tray or your auto-cloner. To provide them with more humidity, you can mist them with some water. If a clone were to die, get rid of it so that it doesn't end up molding and hurting any of your other clones. Your plants are also going to want around 12 hours of light per day.

Most of your clones are going to be ready to transplants in ten to 14 days, but there are some that may take longer. The clones will be ready to be transplanted once the white roots have reached about an inch or two in length.

When the time comes to transplant, you need to make sure that your environment remains sterile, just like you did when taking the cutting. Transplant shock is possible so make sure that you always use gloves when handling them.

To transplant, add soil to the pot. Water your soil before you plant the clone. This will ensure that the soil doesn't move around once the clone has been placed into its new home. After the water has drained away, using two fingers, dig a hole that is about one to two inches deep or just big enough to bury the roots. Carefully place the clone into the dirt and gently cover it with soil.

Your clone should start to flower within the next two to three months if they are planted outside, or after you have switched their lighting up from 18/6 to 12/12 to induce flowering, but it is fine if you want to extend their vegetative stage when they are grown indoors. Make sure you keep a close eye on these plants after they have begun to form flowers. While clones are considered genetic replicas, there is a chance that they could end up becoming hermaphrodites. There are times when a clone may end up growing into the opposite sex of their mother plant because of the stress they are placed under during the cloning process, so don't be shocked if this were to happen to you.

Cloning for Sex

When you want to clone for only females, you will need to take more than one cutting. Make sure that you don't keep the lights on for 12 hours during the day. Instead, you need to make sure that they are deprived of light to help initiate the flowering phase. This should only be done to cuttings that were taken off of plants that were in the third or fourth week of the vegetative state, which you can tell when they develop a calyx.

You will want your plants to have complete, uninterrupted darkness for at least 12 hours each day for a solid two weeks. You have to make sure that this is accomplished correctly because if the light hits them, the process isn't going to work, and you are going to have to start over.

After about two weeks, blossoms will be forming on your new plants, assuming that everything was done right. Let the flowering process continue on until you can spot the female and male plants. Remove the male plants unless you want to use them for seeding, and then transplant your female plants.

In a week after transplanting, your plants should have returned back to the vegetative phases, assuming that they are getting at least 13 hours of light each day. If you don't see any results, try to expose them to 48 straight hours.

Get Them Rooting

Marijuana cuttings tend to root quickly if you keep them in the right condition and if they are prepared right. Until they start to form roots, however, they have a limited ability to maintain water. To make sure they don't cause a water shortage, you have to trim the plants well.

To keep things sterile, boost the water's oxygen content, and encourage the root growth, create a mixture of five parts water to one part of hydrogen peroxide. Let the cuttings have about ten Watts of cold, white fluorescent light for every square foot. You should make sure that your clones are kept in 65% or more humidity. If you are using a cover, take it off after five or six days have passed. Even though you have taken the cover off, make sure the humidity remains high.

After around five days, provide them with some flowering fertilizer. Light wattage should be upped to 20 Watts per square foot. During the next ten days, start increasing the strength of your nutrient mixture by adding some extra growing formula. At the moment you began the process to when you see roots should be around two weeks.

Cuttings From Flowering Plants

If you choose to take a cutting off of a flowering plant, make sure you pick a limb that is in a shaded space so that the buds are less mature then get rid of them. They will die anyway. Make sure that you don't clone a plant that has reached its second week of flowering.

Make sure that you avoid any stems that are woody. Hard stems will make it harder for the roots to form. It is hard to get a cutting from a flowering plant to root, and it will normally take longer to root. During the root process, the plant may end up looking as if it is dying. Give it a day or so before throwing in the towel.

After it has rooted, clones that have been taken from flowering plants will act differently from others, but as long as you keep them in the right amount of light and the correct conditions, it will start to look like a regular plant after a few weeks. When they root successfully, they will often be bushier than the mother plant.

Cloning is able to do wonders for your cannabis garden by saving money and time, and it will ensure that you have a genetically consistent crop. You won't have to have much to get started with the cloning process, and if you do it correctly, you can have a harvest of your most favorite cannabis all year.

CHAPTER 7

FLOWERING

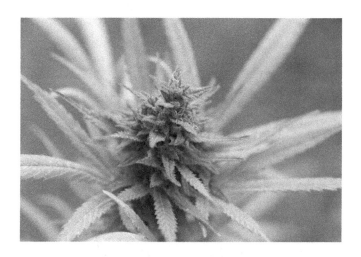

The most important stage you need to understand is the flowering stage. The cannabis plant comes with many different characteristics during its various growing stages, but for most home growers, the last flower stage tends to be the most exciting. The main reason is that this stage will reveal what the quantity and quality of your harvest are going to be like. When you understand this process, it will make it easier to grow.

The flowering stage starts as soon as the vegetative stage has ended. This will normally take about three to four weeks, but it can vary by strain, so make sure that you consider what strain you are growing. If you are growing indoors using photoperiod seeds, the flowering stage will occur when you switch to the 12/12 light schedule. This means that your plant should receive an equal amount of light and dark each day. If you have auto-flowering seeds, then the plant's genetics will decide when this period will start. After the flowering has be-gun, this stage will last around seven to nine weeks. We are going to divide this stage down into sub-stages to help you understand how they grow.

The Flowering Stage: Weeks One to Three

After the plants start to get 12 hours of darkness every day, they will believe that winter is getting close and will start to get ready to produce offspring. This first part of the flowering stage includes a large spurt in its growth to give the plant plenty of size and strength to help sup-port the buds they are getting ready to form. This is so dramatic that a lot of cannabis plants will double or tri-ple in their height at this time.

This is a great time for your plant. At this part of the flowering process, the plants will be very resilient and can recover quickly from problems. This is the same re-siliency that happens during their vegetative growth pe-riod.

During this flowering stage, the plant will begin to move its energy from the vegetative growth into the produc-tion of buds that it thinks is going to make offsprings. Without being pollinated by a male plant, the cannabis plant will use all of the energy it would have used to make seeds for increasing the number and size of buds that normally holds the seeds.

There are some cannabis growers who believe the growth spurt at this time means that it is still going to need the same types of nutrients it used during the vegetative period, like nitrogen. Another idea suggests that introducing nutrients that are needed for bud production, like magnesium and phosphorous, can help to limit how much it stretches and helps to jumpstart the budding by having its nutrients already available. Regardless of your beliefs, the plant should slowly be switched to blooming nutrients at this time.

You will also start to see single leaves starting to bunch on the top of you the colas of every plant. White pistils will come out of the middle of these. This is the first sign of bud production.

If you plan on training your plant, this is when you should start. Low-stress training will involve bending the stems gently so that that it creates a flat canopy. The flat canopy makes sure that there is an even distribution of light to every area of the plant. For outdoor plants, this is not necessary as the sun will naturally pass across their surface. Sections that don't get direct access to light won't produce mature buds and tend to get removed to allow the plant to send more energy to the areas of the plants that do receive a lot of light.

Budlets: Weeks Three to Four

The growth spurt will slow down as the cannabis plant begins to form tiny buds or budlets. Now you have entered into the second leg of the flowering stage. Each new stage of this cycle is more critical than the previous, so be careful since mistakes or problems can hurt your quality or yield.

This time should be used to observe your plants carefully and try to see if there are any signs of problems. One of the easiest signs to see is problems on the leaves. For example, nutrient toxicity will cause the tips of the leaves to turn yellow or brown. If you don't lower how many nutrients you give your plant, this burn will start to spread across the plant, and it can be severely affected. If it does not get treated, your plant won't be able to create food for itself.

Nutrient deficiencies are a lot less detrimental as too many nutrients because you can always add more, but you need to keep track of how you feed them and adjust it as soon as you figure out what your problem is. The plants will still be able to recover to some extent, but it is always better to make sure that you don't have any problems.

You will also see that some of the leaves on the bottom of the plant will turn yellow around this time. If there are only a few leaves that do this, don't worry. It is normal for a few of these leaves to yellow if they aren't getting enough light. The plant is taking all of the nutrients out of those leaves to keep the buds that are developing, growing. Plants are very smart. They don't like to waste resources on things that aren't productive.

Fattening Buds: Weeks Four to Six

The next part of the flowering process is the fattening up of the budlets. The tiny buds will start to grow quickly. This happens rapidly, and you are still going to see the pistils sticking out of them.

The growth spurt has pretty much stopped by this point, so you don't really need to continue training your plant. The plant is completely focused on its bud production. However, you can continue to do a bit of training if you find that the canopy of your plants is not flat enough. Remember, training at this time can be very risky. Unlike during the growth spurt, any training that is performed now causes a lot of stress to the plant since its vegetative growth has stopped. The plant may recover but do your best to avoid this type of training because it can slow the bud fattening process.

Since your plant isn't going to grow any more leaves, do what you can to preserve the ones that it has. First, make sure it gets the right amount of nutrients so that it doesn't get burned or experience a deficiency. Second, give them enough water since transpiration is going to pick up. Excess stress from the improper amount of light, heat, or humidity can cause the leaves to yellow and fall off.

You should not try to get rid of any leaves unless you are very experienced in this process and can strategically remove the right leaves that will help to expose more bud sites.

You will want to maintain as many leaves as you need to in order to have a full canopy because if you take off too many at the point, your plant won't have enough foliage to absorb the light it needs to maximize yields. However, if you have a lot of healthy leaves, there will be a "reserve" of leaves that can help the plant to do well and remain healthy. During this time, most of the pistils will stay white, which means that the buds will continue to get bigger and dense every day.

Ripening of Buds: Weeks Six to Eight

Once the buds begin to ripen, you have moved into the next flowering stage. Any vegetative growth has stopped altogether at this point, and all of the plant's energy is being devoted to the final stages of life. The buds will grow to its largest during this time, which is the reason why you should not use nutrients that help to promote vegetative growth.

Nutrients such as nitrogen are counterproductive at this time because they are not being used in the same amounts now as they were during the vegetative growth. This will create an accumulation in the leaves, which can negatively affect the bud quality after harvest. If there is too much nitrogen present, the plant can become stressed and revert to its vegetative growth or it will self-pollinate and produce seeds.

For some plants, the bottom leaves will start to turn yellow and fall off at this time while others started losing their leaves between weeks four to six. Nevertheless, you will need to be vigilant to make sure that you don't mistake a problem for normal leaf loss. If everything is as it needs to be, your plant should be green and full, with only a few of its bottom leaves discolored.

During this time, you might start to notice that buds form beneath or on the sides of existing buds. This is what is called "fox tailing," and while it naturally occurs in some strains, it is most commonly a sign of environmental stress, either from high temps or too much light. Figure out which could be the reason why you are experiencing it and adjust it.

For example, if your plants ended up growing taller than you thought they would and are close to the grow lights, then you probably need to raise the lights up so that the lights don't burn them. Or, if you have an area of your grow room that is hotter than another, then you should increase the airflow so that the heat can be moved out efficiently.

Too much light or heat can burn or bleach the buds. They will lose some of their potency since the evaporation will cause your plant to lose a bit of its cannabinoids.

End of Flowering: Week Eight+

The exact week, when you will get to harvest, is going to depend on what strain you have. The harvest window is normally about a week-long, and that the THC will start to turn into CBN, which isn't as potent and causes you to feel sleepy. Close to the end of flowering, the pistils, on most strains, will turn orange. This lets you know that new buds are not being grown, and harvest time is getting close. The trichomes will switch from clear to milky as they increase the THC, and will start to change to an amber color, which tells you that the THC is degrading to CBN. Both of the phases tend to overlap a bit, but most growers think that plants reach the full potency when around five to 30 percent of the trichomes have turned amber in color and the rest are still milky.

You have to be careful at this point. They are super sensitive to all kinds of conditions at the end of the growing season. If they don't have enough airflow, excess moisture can get trapped in the buds, which can cause them to rot, which will spread and destroy the rest of the harvest.

It is very common for a few buds to become heavier than what their branch can hold. You may have to make some support for them so that they remain upright. There are plenty of tools for this.

The end of the growing cycle will bring about the common "weed" smell. You should expect this to reach overpowering levels. Don't be all that surprised if your visitors or neighbors start to ask you about the smells drifting out of your house. If you exhaust your air through a carbon filter can help to manage the odor.

Shortly before harvesting, you need to flush the plants. Flushing is simply when you stop giving your plants their nutrients and start giving them pH-appropriate water. You need to flush them for a couple of days to a week, depending on how long your plant's flowering stage is and the growing medium you used. Soil tends to retain more nutrients than soilless mediums, so it is going to need a longer flush.

Flushing helps to give the plant a chance to use all the nutrients that you have in the system so that it doesn't affect its smell and taste. Flushing also gets rid of salts that may have built up in the growing medium. Basically, it gives you one last chance to improve its quality.

The flowering stage is the most rewarding stage, and if you fully understand this process, the more you will be able to gain from it. There are five distinct parts to the flowering stage, each with their own needs and characteristics. Proper oversight of these stages helps to place you firmly on the path to having the biggest and most potent buds to harvest.

You also have to take into consideration the strain you are growing. There will be tweaks you will need to make, depending on what you are growing. And if you are using auto-flowering strains, you will still notice that they go through these stages as well. The main difference is the fact that they will reach their flowering stage no matter what light they have experienced.

CHAPTER 8
HARVESTING

———————— ◆◇◆ ————————

Knowing when to harvest your marijuana is the hardest aspect of growing marijuana. If you harvest it too soon, it isn't going to be potent enough. If you wait too long, you will have marijuana that has an extremely strong taste and will be too narcotic.

Even though harvesting can be tricky, there are some tips and strategies that will help you know when the time is right for harvesting. This chapter will explain the different methods for figuring out when your plants are ready to be harvested and what to expect during the process.

Basics of Harvesting

Marijuana harvesting is a lot like harvesting other fruits. The more you wait, the stronger the alcohol and the grapes will taste better. When you are growing marijuana, if you wait for longer, you will get more cannabinoids.

This basically means you will have a stronger product.

Once the plant has flowered, it will begin to die. There are several signs that will tell you that this event is about to happen like:

- Leaves beginning to turn yellow and dying
- The resin on the buds getting dark and turning brown
- Stems getting broader
- Pistils turning red

If your plants have flowered and you see any of these signs, you are probably ready to begin harvesting. There are some guidelines about when to harvest, but most growers will argue about when the "best" time is. It is just like other vegetables and fruits; it all depends on what you like the best.

When to Harvest

There are several ways to figure out the best time to harvest. We will go over them in more details in a bit, but this will give you an idea:

- Trichomes
  o If the trichomes are amber-colored, the plants are too ripe
  o If the trichomes are between a milky white and amber, perfect for harvesting
  o If the trichomes are clear, you need to wait

- Pistils

o 90 to 100 percent brown, the marijuana will have a heavy and sharp taste

o 70 to 90 percent brown, the marijuana will have a heavy, ripe taste

o 50 to 70 percent brown, the marijuana is too young and will have a very light taste

- Flowering Time

o Autoflowering – ten weeks from seedling to budding

o Sativa – ready to harvest after it has flowered for ten weeks

o Indica – ready to harvest after it has flowered for eight weeks

Trichomes and Pistils

You will need to have some sort of magnifying tool for this part. This is the best way to see if marijuana is ready to be harvested.

How can you know it is the right time?

You will need to look for trichomes that are filled with resin. They will be glistening with the resin.

If you have a good magnifying tool, you will be able to see these details clearly. Here are some magnifying tools to think about:

- Digital Microscope

These are a bit expensive, but they are the best option because they will give you a clear view of your plants. The biggest downside is you are going to need a laptop with you to see your results. If you do decide to get one, you need to take the time to read through the instructions.

- Handheld Magnifying Tools

This option is good, but they can be a bit cumbersome to use. You have to get the focus just right in order to see your trichomes.

- Jewelers Loupe

This one is perfect if you are on a tight budget. It isn't all that great, but it will give you a bit of a gauge to see your plants up close.

Just remember that any of these will let you see the trichomes, but if you don't know how to use them right, they aren't going to help you.

Longer Isn't Better

Even though letting your plants flower for longer might give you a bigger harvest, it might not give you the best results. You have to time it just right.

I cannot express this enough:

If you let your plants flower too long, you might experience an unpleasant and overpowering flavor. You might experience some decreased effectiveness in the THC.

The best way to not reach this point is to watch the pistil color closely. This is the most common way to know when to harvest.

There are some growers who will harvest their plants as soon as the pistils start turning red. While others will wait until they are completely red, and the resin turns dark.

As stated earlier, you can look at the resin of your plants to see if they are at the harvesting stage. When you look at them through a magnifying glass, the glands will be covered in resin and enlarged when they are mature. They might even swell out and look a bit deformed.

This is when you need to harvest.

The resin is going to turn darker. It will change from being transparent to an opaque amber when it matures. You need to harvest once the resin is transparent and sticky. When the resin gets darker and turns more of an amber color, there isn't a lot of time left before the THC begins to deteriorate.

Basing Harvest on Flowering Time

Looking at the flowers is only one way to know if you need to harvest. You could just time it based on the flowering time of the plant. Basically, all marijuana plants will be ready for harvest at about the same time. There are some variations based on certain strains. You will need to know all about your strain to be able to use this method the right way.

Successful growers will do these things before they start timing their harvest:

- Read all comments from other growers
- Read the entire description of the strain

If you bought your seeds from a reputable source, somebody has already shared some ideas about when it will be ready to harvest. There are other variables that can impact when your plants will be ready to harvest. One condition is your grow room or outdoor climate. These can play huge roles in your plant's development.

So, basically, there isn't any way to accurately decide when you need to harvest. There are a few guidelines that will give you the idea that the time is right.

Indica Plants Harvesting Time

If you grow Indica plants, the flowering time will last about eight weeks before they will be ready for harvest. If you grow your plants outdoors, they should be ready to harvest close to the end of September.

Sative Plants Harvesting Time

If you grow Sativa plants, the flowering time will last about 12 weeks. With that being said, there are several strains that will flower faster. These will only flower for about nine to ten weeks. Remember to read its description before you buy them to be sure. Sativas are normally ready to be harvested by the end of October.

Autoflowering Plants Harvesting Time

Autoflowering plants don't rely on the changes in lighting. This makes them a bit easier to predict just using flowering time. When you see the very first seedling, you will know you can harvest in ten weeks.

Even though basing your harvest on the plants flowering time isn't exact, it is a good point to help you figure out when you should harvest your marijuana plants. This also will work to your advantage to help you plan ahead since you will be able to see what your season might look like.

Be On the Look Out for Brown or Red Pistils

Looking closely at the pistils is the easiest and best method to help you decide when you need to harvest. Look at the bud's pistils to see what color they are. If they are white, it is way too early to harvest. If they are red or brown, you have missed the best time, and you need to harvest immediately before the THC lowers any more.

If you want to use this method, here are some tips to follow:

- If zero to 49 percent of the plant's pistils are brown, they aren't ready for harvest.

- If 50 to 75 percent of the pistils are brown, harvest time is close. It is still a bit early. If you harvest now, they will have a mellower high and a light taste. You can wait just a bit longer.

- If 70 to 90 percent of the pistils are brown, harvest your plants now. They are as heavy and strong as they are ever going to be.

- If 90 to 100 percent of the pistils are brown, you have missed your harvest. Their taste is going to be very heavy and will have a narcotic effect. You have to harvest right now.

Are My Plants Ready?

I know it is hard to wait when the pistils begin changing colors, but you have to. Here is why:

When the pistils are about two-thirds brown, you will be able to harvest them safely.

If you aren't sure you want to do the 70 to 90 percent brown, just experiment and see for yourself. There are some new growers who harvest their plants at various times during the flowering stage so they can figure out when is the best time for their personal preference. Remember that some people like to harvest their marijuana earlier because it has a lighter and more uplifting effect. Other people want theirs as potent as they can get it.

The time that you harvest is going to affect the quality of the buds. What you consider as "high-quality" is all about your personal taste. You have to decide for yourself. The best thing about growing marijuana is you have the ability to control this powerful variable.

Look at Your Trichomes

If watching the pistils didn't work for you and you have some of the magnification tools above, you can look at the trichomes to figure out if your plants are ready to harvest. This method is considered the most accurate, so it would be a good idea to know what you are looking for.

This concept is very simple; you just look at the trichomes on your buds. These grow on the buds, and they look like little mushrooms because that will have a ball on top. Some of these trichomes are resin glands. They are going to have a crystalline structure or they might look frosty while growing on the buds and leaves of the plant.

Why is this important?

Trichomes are responsible for marijuana's stickiness. They are where most of the THC and chemicals get housed. If you harvest based on trichomes, you will figure out when the trichomes are at the highest TCH level. This is hard to see with your naked eye.

How to Harvest Based on Trichomes

How will you know that your trichomes are ready? You have to compare them with these guidelines:

- White, Clear Hairs

This is not the right time to harvest. When the trichomes are very clear, they aren't potent enough to be harvested. Your final yield is going to suffer. You need to wait until almost half of the hairs are a dark color and aren't standing out straight.

- Cloudy, Half Clear Trichomes

This means it is still too soon to harvest your plants. The buds haven't gotten to their whole potential even though they will still give you a high if you did harvest at this point. The high you will get will be more energetic. You will get a better flavor and odor if you wait just a bit longer.

- Very Cloudy Trichomes

Great, you have reached the best time for harvesting your plants. Your buds are going to have the highest THC levels. If you would like to maximize your yield, you have to act fast. You will know the plants have reached this point when 50 to 70 percent of the hairs aren't white anymore.

Let me repeat myself:

You have to harvest your buds right now. Your plants are at their most potent levels right now. Because of this, the high you will get from these buds will give you some serious pain relief and euphoria. This will be the most intense high you are able to get.

- Cloudy, Amber Trichomes

If you let your plants get this far, it is after their peak THC levels. This happens because the buds have less TCH and more CBN. If you want a more anxiety-reducing, relaxing high, this is the best time to harvest your buds.

Any high you get from the marijuana that was harvested during this time will be more narcotic and will result in a "couchlock" effect. This stage is reached when 70 to 90 percent of the hairs have turned dark.

In terms of figuring out the perfect time to harvest, try to experiment with your harvest times to get the results you are after. Harvesting some buds during their peak time and then save some to harvest after they have matured a bit longer. By doing this, you will have many different options.

When you harvest, you have to remember to label every single thing. You don't want to get a relaxed high when you really wanted a more energetic high.

Ready to Harvest

Before you start harvesting, you need to have these things handy:

- Gloves

- A bowl of isopropyl alcohol

- Heavy-duty shears

You will use the shears to cut through the plant's base. You will use the alcohol to clean your hands and tools because the resin is super sticky. It would be best if you used gloves while cutting the plants because it can get very messy.

So, you have decided that your plants are ready to be harvested. You will begin by getting rid of the grow lamps in your growing room. You will need to hang some wire from the ceiling as you will need this for your plants.

Carefully cut the plant at the base. You will hang it upside down from the wires hanging from the ceiling. Turn on fans and aim it underneath the buds. Try to keep the humidity in the room to about 45 percent. The temperature should be able 64 degrees. The room needs to be dark and keep the extractor fan running.

After you have cut your plants and hung them upside down, now you just need to wait until all the excess moisture has gone out of them. It has to evaporate from the plants while the chlorophyll in the plants breaks down. Don't try to do this too fast because it could cause some chlorophyll to stay inside, and this will change the taste of your marijuana. This is why the room needs to have moderate temperatures and stay dark.

The drying stage could last anywhere from form ten to 14 days. You will need to keep a close eye on them while they are drying. Look for mold. You have to make sure that no mold is growing on your plants. This is why you need to keep the humidity very low, and the temperature stays the same.

Harvesting Outdoors

It doesn't matter if you grew your marijuana inside or out, your plants will show you when they are ready to be harvested.

Other than looking at their pistils and trichomes, you need to think about the weather. You will need to harvest them outside when it is a calm and dry day. Nobody really likes harvesting anything when it is raining.

When looking at your plant, you need to pay attention to the buds and leaves. The main characteristics of the plant are going to change a lot, and this will let you know that it is time.

The plant's larger leaves are going to turn a yellowish-brown color, and this shows that the plant is slowly dying. The stigmas are going to wither at the bud's base while it is still a white color on its top.

The color of the buds is another indicator that it is time to harvest. It would be good to pick them when they begin losing their rich green color.

When you get ready to harvest your outdoor plants, begin by gathering some sealable bags. If you use zip-top bags, make sure you have a dark bag with you too since zip-top bags are transparent.

Cut the plants into lengths that you can easily transport. Cut the stalks so that they can fit into your bags. Be sure you don't spend too much time at your site when you are harvesting. You need to be fast but efficient. Remember that the important thing is removing your plants and transporting them safely. The way you do this is up to you.

When you do harvest outdoors, you need to do it before the first frost can damage your plants. Harvest on a nice day that has lots of sun and clear skies. Don't try to overthink this, because harvesting in the rain isn't going to be the end of the world.

Rain is going to increase the drying time just a bit, but it won't have any effects on the resin glands and buds. Never relax until you have arrived home safe with your plants after you are home, you won't have to worry about much from this point.

CHAPTER 9

DRYING AND CURING

◆ ◇ ◆

Growing marijuana doesn't stop when you harvest it. Drying and curing your marijuana needs to be done properly so that your stash is free from contamination and mold. These procedures will create a better high, and the buds will taste better.

After you have watched your plants grow and flower, it is time to collect your plants. Before you can enjoy smoking your homegrown marijuana, you are going to need to dry and cure your marijuana.

After you have worked for months tending to your plants and you finally got to harvest a good crop of fragrant buds that you are just dying to try, you have to wait until they have dried out first. Even though you might be tempted to dry the buds as fast as possible, curing is a process of getting the moisture from the plants under environmental conditions that are perfect so that you will have a better product.

Curing Marijuana the Right Way Will Increase Its Potency

Marijuana plants will produce cannabinoids and THCA or tetrahydrocannabinolic acid through biosynthesis. This is when specific compounds get converted gradually into new blends. THCA then gets turned into the main compound in THC.

This process won't stop completely right when you cut down the plants. If you keep your harvested marijuana in a temperature that is between 60 and 70 degrees while the humidity stays at about 45 to 55 percent, the conversion of the non-psychoactive cannabinoids into THCA will keep going, and the buds will get more potent. Drying the marijuana in dry, warm conditions stops this process faster.

Curing Can Change the Quality and Flavor

Most of the aromatic compounds that give marijuana its unique flavor and smell are very volatile. It can evaporate and degrade at temperatures below 70 degrees. Curing slow and low will keep the terpenes faster than a hot, quick drying process.

These kinds of conditions will create the best environment for aerobic bacteria and enzymes to break down any leftover sugars and minerals that get produced by chlorophyll decomposing while it dries. When the leftover minerals and sugars are present, this is what creates the throat-burning, harsh sensations when you smoke marijuana that hasn't been cured properly.

Curing Will Preserve Your Marijuana

Curing your marijuana properly will allow you to store it for a long time without worrying about it losing its THC content or molding. Buds that have been cured well can be kept in an airtight container in a dark, cool place for two years without any potency being lost.

Curing and Drying Your Marijuana

There are various ways you can cure your marijuana. Most people will use a variation of a popular method. Even though you can freeze-dry it, cure it using dry ice, and water cure it, we will be focusing on the best and easiest way to get the best out of your harvest.

Initial Drying

The way you do this step all depends on the way you harvest your marijuana. The way most people do it is to cut the branches between 12 and 16 inches long and get rid of any leaves that you don't want. You will then hang the branches from a wire or string. There are some growers who will cut the entire plant, and others will just cut the buds from the branches and put them on drying racks. You could completely manicure the flowers before you dry them or you can wait until after they have dried.

It doesn't really matter which method you use; you need to keep the harvested marijuana in a dark room with the humidity between 45 and 55 percent and the temperature between 60 and 70 degrees. You also need a small fan to keep the air circulating. This is critical to keep the aroma and flavor of the buds. It would be ideal to have an air conditioning unit, dehumidifier, or another way to make sure the conditions in the room stay stable.

Once your flowers feel crunchy on the outside, and the tiny branches snap when bent, you are ready to move to the next step. This all depends on the flowers' density and the conditions of the environment; it could take between five and 15 days for this drying stage to be done.

Final Cure .

When you have figured out that your buds are mostly dry, now it is time to cure them. There are several steps to this process:

1. You will need to manicure the buds and remove them from the branches if you haven't done this already.

2. Put the trimmed buds into an airtight container. Wide mouth quart canning jars the used the most. You could use plastic, wood, metal, or ceramic containers, too. Some people like using zip-top bags. These are fine, but plastic bags aren't suitable for curing because they don't keep oxygen out and this can degrade if they come in contact with specific terpenes that are

found in marijuana. Pack your buds loosely in the containers. Fill them to the top but don't compact them down or crush the buds.

3. Seal your container and put them in a dark, dry, cool spot to finish this process. You will notice on the first day that your buds aren't crunchy and dry on the outside because the moisture from the inside of the flowers is rehydrating the outside. If this isn't happening, you over-dried your marijuana.

4. Within the first week, open your containers many times during the day to allow the flowers to breathe for several minutes. This lets moisture escape and will replenish the oxygen in the container. If you notice an ammonia-like odor coming from your container, this means that the buds aren't dry enough to be cured, and anaerobic bacteria are eating them. This will cause rotten, moldy marijuana. Once the first week is over, you only need to open the container every couple of days.

After your marijuana has been in containers for two to three weeks, it will be cured enough to give a good experience. If you leave them between four and eight weeks, it will improve them more. There are some strains that need to be cured for six months.

This process is probably what most people overlook when they grow marijuana. This process was ignored during the time that the "black market" was our only way to get marijuana. Because of the competition in the recreational and medical markets, most growers pay attention to this process that will turn a good product into a really excellent one. You can do the same thing with what you grow at home.

FAQs

Here are the answers to the most asked questions about drying and curing marijuana, so you can maximize the potency and flavor of your buds.

- What is the difference between curing and drying?

Drying is just that drying out the fresh buds so they don't have as much moisture so they can be vaporized or smoked properly. Curing involves storing the buds in airtight containers for at least two weeks. This will help develop the aroma and flavor of the buds while they mature.

- How long does it take to cure marijuana?

Most growers cure their weed for about one month, but curing for two months will get the most aroma and flavor from your buds.

- Why does marijuana need to be dried and cured?

Curing is very important since it can help to preserve your marijuana so you can store it for a long amount of time while it keeps its potency and flavor. After you have harvested your marijuana, they will have a lot of starch and sugar in them that can be attacked by enzymes and airborne bacteria. When you cure the buds, you are encouraging the degradation of those nutrients, which makes it a better tasting, smoother smoke.

- How do I store the buds after they have been cured and dried?

After you have cured your buds, you can keep them in the same jar. Just place them in a dry, dark, cool space. You won't have to check on them as often. Just make sure to keep the sealed to keep them from drying out too much. If you have lots of marijuana, you could invest in a humidity pack or something like it to keep them fresh for longer periods of time.

- How to cure buds?

If you decided to trim the buds while they were wet, you can move on to the curing stage once they have dried. If you trimmed them dry, you will need to do this before you move to the curing process.

When the buds have been trimmed and dried, put them in a wide-mouthed jar. Fill the jar about three-quarters full so that you have room for air. This reduces the risk of mildew or mold ruining your buds. When you have filled your jars, place them in a dark, dry environment. You will need to check them every single day for two weeks.

While you are doing this, leave the jars open for a little while. Look at every bud to see if you see any signs of mold. If you do find a bud that has been infected, remove it, so the fungus doesn't spread.

When you are constantly checking your buds, it pulls excess moisture from the jars and lets fresh air get to your buds. After two weeks have passed, you can begin enjoying your marijuana, but if you wait longer, it will taste better.

- How will I know my buds have been dried properly and are ready to be cured?

There is a very simple test that will tell you if your buds are dry enough. Just take a tiny branch and bend it. If it snaps in two, they are dry enough to move to the curing process. If the branch only bends, they need to dry for a longer time.

- How long will it take to dry the buds properly?

There are several factors that can affect how long it will take for your marijuana to dry. How large your buds are will the drying time because denser, larger buds are going to take longer to dry than small ones. The way you trim your plants also come into play. You have to remember that branches hold more water, so if you hang the larger branches, they are going to take longer to dry than individual buds or small branches. The airflow, humidity, and temperature in the drying space will impact the time it will take to dry the marijuana.

Basically, the drying process will take between seven and 12 days. It all depends on the factors above. During this process, the buds are going to lose lots of water.

This means they are going to lose weight and shrink in size.

- Once the buds have been harvested and trimmed, how is the best way to dry them?

If you want your buds to dry evenly, you will need to make sure that air can move around them freely. This means they need to feel the air on all sides. The best way you can do this is by hanging your trimmed and cut branches on either string or wire. If you just harvested the buds, you can use a wire rack. You will need to flip your buds to make sure they don't get flattened on one side.

For the best results, you need to hang or position the buds in a dark room that has great air circulation and a humidity level of around 45 to 55 percent.

- What's the best way to trim your marijuana plants?

There are two ways to trim your buds during harvest. Wet trimming means you trim the buds right after harvest. When you dry trim, you will trim the buds after they have dried but before you cure them. I personally like trimming the buds when they are wet. It is easier and more precise, and you won't lose any resin like you do when you handle buds that have been dried. Dry trimming can be a great manicured product that is worthy of being placed on a shelf because it looks so good.

CHAPTER 10

GROWING INDOORS

◆ ◇ ◆

You've decided you want to grow your own marijuana at home. Before you begin working your green thumb, know that growing marijuana inside does have some challenges for new growers. The amount of information you will find on the internet about this subject can overwhelm you. In this chapter, this easy guide will help you get started.

There are several benefits to growing your marijuana inside:

- Security and privacy: Even in states where marijuana is legal, you probably want to make sure your crops are hidden from thieves and nosy neighbors. Growing your plants inside will let you grow them secretly behind locked doors.

- Multiple harvests: When you grow inside, you aren't at the whim of the seasons and sun. You can also allow them to grow as much or as little as you want. You can make the flower when you want to. This allows you to harvest them and then begin another batch immediately. You have the ability to grown anytime you want. This means you can grow during winter.

- Adaptability: If you live in a small house or an apartment, you can still grow marijuana. You have the ability to grow your plants anywhere you have some extra space. Even people who have a small backyard or not a lot of space can do it.

- High-quality plants: Even though it tends to be resource-intensive, growing your plants indoors gives you control over everything in their environment. You have the ability to dial in on the setup that is going to give you the best marijuana.

Find Your Growing Space

The first thing you need to do is set up a growing space for your marijuana. You don't need a whole room to do this. You can use a closet, cabinet, corner of an unfinished basement, tent, or a spare room. Remember that you will need to make sure your plants and equipment fit in the space.

Begin small. When you are first undertaking a growing project, you will want to keep things small for many reasons:

- Any mistakes you make won't cost you a lot of money

- It is easier to take care of a few plants than a greenhouse full

- The smaller the growing area, the less expensive it will be to set up

Keep in mind that you will have some setbacks. You will lose some plants due to disease or pests. Losing two plants won't cost you as much as losing hundreds.

Think big. When you are figuring out your growing space, you are going to want to think about how much room your plants are going to need. You have to think about the fans, ducting, lights, and any other equipment you are going to need. You also need to leave the room so you can work. Marijuana plants will easily double in size in their first few growing stages. You need to be sure you have enough headspace.

If you are growing in a closet, tent, or cabinet, you have the ability to just open it up, take the plants out, and do what you need to do. If not, just make sure you have plenty of elbow room.

Stay clean. You have to be sure that your space can be sanitized easily. You have to keep everything clean when you are growing indoors. You should make sure you have surfaces that are easy to clean. Raw wood, drapes, and carpeting are very hard to clean, so keep away from these materials if at all possible.

Another critical component for a growing room is to make sure it is light tight. If any light leaks into the space during the dark periods, it could confuse the plants and cause them to turn hermaphroditic.

When you are making a decision about where to grow your plants, keep these things in mind:

- Stealth: you will want to keep what you are growing from your nosy neighbors and thieves. Make sure you find a place where fans aren't going to get any unwanted attention.

- Humidity and temperature problems: If the space you chose to grow your plants is very humid and warm, you are going to have problems controlling the environment. Find a dry, cool area that has access to outdoor fresh air.

- Convenience: You are going to have to watch your plants very carefully. Check on them daily is very important. If you are a beginner, you will want to check on them many times during the day until you have everything dialed in. If you have problems getting to your growing room, this step is going to be very hard.

Plants Need Air

Plants have to have fresh air and carbon dioxide in order to grow. This is essential for photosynthesis. You are going to have to make sure that you have a good stream of air moving into and out of your room at all times. This can be achieved by using exhaust fans put at the top of the room to get rid of the warm air. You will need a filtered air inlet on the other side of the room close to the floor.

You will need to make sure that the temperature in the room stays between 70 and 85 degrees when the lights are on. It needs to stay between 58 and 70 degrees when the lights are off. Some strains of marijuana like cooler temperatures whole other like higher temperatures.

How large your exhaust fans need to be depends on how large your grow space is and how much heat your lights give off. HID systems give off tons of heat, especially if you don't have them connected to a hood that is cooled. If you live somewhere where it stays warm most of the year, you can run your light during the night to keep the temperatures in your grow room down.

It would be best to set up the light and run them for some time to figure out the amount of airflow you are going to need to make sure that your plants are kept at a comfortable temperature. This means you can pick out an exhaust fan that is going to give you what you need. If the smell of marijuana plants that are blooming bothers you, add charcoal filters to the exhaust fan.

You can come up with a sealed and artificial environment through the use of a supplemental CO_2 system, dehumidifier, and air conditioner. These can be very expensive, and it isn't recommended if you are a first-time grower.

You should always have a constant breeze flowing through your grow room because it helps to strengthen the plant's stems and will create an environment that will prevent flying pests and mod. A simple wall mount fan that circulates works well. You shouldn't point the fan directly at your plants because this can cause wind-burn.

Choose Your Monitors and Controllers

When you have selected your climate control equipment and lights, you will need to automate their functions. These can be expensive and sophisticated, but they can control the CO2 levels, humidity levels, temperature, and lights. You will need to make sure that you have a 24-hour timer for your lights as well as a thermostat switch you can adjust to work your exhaust fan.

The most important thing about growing marijuana is correctly controlling the light and dark phases. While in a vegetative state, you want to make sure that they are exposed to at least 18 hours of light. You can switch to 12 hours of light when you are ready for them to bloom. You will need to be able to turn the lights off and on at the same time daily, or you will stress your plants. You need a timer for this. You may want to have a timer on your exhaust fan as well, but make sure that you go with one of the more expensive options because you tend to get what you pay for.

When it comes to a thermostat switch, you simply set the thermostat to the highest temperature you would want in the growing space and then plug the timer into the fan. If the temperature of the room hits above that set temperature, it will trigger the exhaust fan to turn on until the temperature drops below that set temp. This will save you energy while maintaining a regular temperature.

Because you aren't going to spend a lot of time within that growing room, having a combination thermostat and hygrometer with a low and high memory is very helpful to keep a watch on the condition of your grow room. These inexpensive, small devices show you the current humidity and temperature levels, but the lowest and highest reading for the time since you checked it last.

Choose a Container

The container you pick out is going to depend greatly on the size of your plants, system, and medium. The ebb-and-flow hydroponic system that uses small net pots that are filled with rockwool or clay pebbles is good to use when you want to grow a lot of plants at one time. A system called "super-soil" grows a large plant in a ten-gallon nursery pot.

There are some inexpensive options that use cloth bags or disposable, perforated plastic bags that you can use to enhance the airflow in the grow room. Other people like using "smart pots." Most first time growers will grow their first plant in a five-gallon bucket.

You need to make sure that your marijuana plants have lots of drainage as they are very sensitive to sitting in water or having "wet feet." If you choose to reuse your containers, you should make sure that some holes have been drilled into the bottom, and they are placed into trays.

CHAPTER 11
GROWING INDOORS: LIGHTING AND SOIL

———————— ◆ ◇ ◆ ————————

The next step in setting up an indoor cannabis garden is to pick out the best lighting and soil. Lighting is one of the most crucial aspects of growing cannabis. Unless you are using auto-flowering plants, your cannabis plants won't start producing flowers until it receives a certain amount of daylight and darkness. That means you have to make sure you have a good quality grow light.

Choosing Grow Lights

The number one environmental factor that can hurt your yields is the quality of light you have for your plants, so it is best to pick out the best setup that you are able to afford. We'll quickly go over some of the most common types of grow lights that you can use.

- HID Grow Lights

HID, or high-intensity discharge, lights are the ones that most people will use due to the fact they are very efficient, both cost-wise and electricity-wise. Their cost is more than fluorescent or incandescent lights, but they give off more light per the amount of electricity they use. On the flip side, they aren't as efficient as LEDs, but they cost a tenth for comparable units.

There are two types of HID lamps. Metal halide produces a blue-ish white light and should be used during the vegetative phase. The other HID light, high-pressure sodium, produces a red-orange light and is often used during the flowering phase.

Besides the bulbs, HID setups will need a hood/reflector and a ballast for every light. There are some ballasts designed for HPS lamps and some for MH lamps, while some newer ones can run both.

If you are unable to afford both of these bulbs to start, you can just get the HPS light because they produce more light. The magnetic ballast is more cost-efficient, but they run hotter, aren't as efficient, and the bulbs to it are harder to find. A digital ballast tends to work better, but they do cost more. Keep an eye out for cheap ballasts as they aren't well shielded and can end up creating electromagnetic interferences that can harm your WiFi and radio signals

Unless your grow room is very large and open with a lot of ventilation, you will have to make sure that you use an air-cooled hood that your lights are mounted in because HID bulbs let off quite a bit of heat. This is where the use of an exhaust fan comes in and is going to add more to your initial cost to get things started.

- Fluorescent Grow Lights

Hobby growers like to use the fluorescent light fixture fixed with a T5 bulb because they are cheaper, and everything that you are going to need comes in the lighting package. You also aren't going to need to have a cooling system with these lights because they don't generate a lot of heat.

The biggest issue with them is that they aren't as efficient as other options and don't produce as much light per watt. Space tends to be a concern as well since you are going to need 19 four-foot bulbs to match the output of a 600 watt HPS

- LED Lights

The technology or LED lights has been around for a long time, but it has only been during the past few years that it has been created to work as an efficient grow light fixture. The biggest problem is the upfront cost of LED lights. Some of the best setups can end up costing you ten times what an HID setup cost you. The benefits, though, last a lot longer, they don't use as much electricity, create a lot less heat, and they are made to generate a fuller light spectrum light, which can help your plants grow better.

Unfortunately, there are a lot of shoddy lights out on the market that is marketed towards first-time growers, so make sure that you do some research and read reviews before you purchase them.

- Induction Lights

Induction lamps, which are also called electrodeless fluorescents, is an old technology that has been adapted for indoor growers. It was created in the late 1800s by Nikola Tesla. They have more efficiency and last longer than the regular fluorescent light. The main issue is its availability and price.

Figure Out Your Growing Medium

When you grow marijuana indoors, this means that you have various media you can choose from and whether a pot full of soil or using hydroponics with some rockwool would be better. Every medium will have its own unique drawbacks and benefits. Let's look at the most popular ways and the media they use.

- Hydroponics or Soilless

People who are growing marijuana indoors are beginning to use a hydroponic system for growing marijuana plants. This way requires you to feed them solutions that are concentrated that is full of nutrients that get absorbed directly into the roots.

This technique leads to faster growth and larger yields. It also requires more precisions since plants are faster to react to under or overfeeding and are susceptible to burn and nutrient lockdown.

Various materials that are used include coco coir, perlite, clay pebbles, vermiculite, and rockwool. You can find soilless mixes that combine two or more of these options to make a better growing mixture. You can use the options in a hydroponic system or can also use them in a planter.

- Regular Soil

The most traditional medium for growing marijuana indoors is soil. It is also the most forgiving, which makes it the best option for the beginner grower. You can use pretty much any quality potting mixture. The one thing you should make sure you don't use is something that contains artificial fertilizers that have extended-release formulas such as "Miracle-Gro." You absolutely can't grow good marijuana with this.

The best choice for beginners would be to use an organic pre-fertilized soil, which is often referred to as a "supersoil." This soil is able to easily grow marijuana plants all throughout the growing process without the need for added nutrients, as long as you use it correctly. You can make this yourself by combining bat guano, worm castings, along with other composted material and great soil, then let it sit for a few weeks to combine. You could also buy it from various suppliers.

Just like with all other organic growing media, you are going to have to use bacteria and mycorrhizae in the soil to speed up the organic matter being turned into nutrients that can be used by the plant. You could use a normal soil mix and then add liquid nutrients when the soil becomes depleted.

CHAPTER 12

GROWING INDOORS: WATER AND NUTRIENTS

—————— ◆◇◆ ——————

The last two things you are going to have to consider when it comes to growing your plants indoors is watering and nutrients. Both of these are important factors in making sure that your plants grow to their full maturity and produce the buds you want. Even if grown outdoors, water and nutrients tend to be the two aspects that have to be monitored and dealt with the most.

Making Sure Your Cannabis is Fed

Making sure that you grow high-quality cannabis flowers is going to require more fertilizer, or nutrients than your average garden crop. Your plant is going to feed off of three main nutrients, which are also called macronutrients:

- Potassium (K)

- Phosphorus (P)

- Nitrogen (N)

They will also need smaller quantities of micronutrients, such as:

- Copper

- Iron

- Magnesium

- Calcium

If you don't decide to use a pre-fertilized organic soil mixture, you will need to make sure that your plants are given nutrients at least once per week using the correct solution. You can find the nutrients solutions sold in concentrated liquids or powders that are supposed to be mixed with water. They are typically formulated to be used during the vegetative or flowering phase. They have separate mixtures for these phases because the plant's macronutrient requirements will change throughout its growing life. Cannabis has to have a lot of nitrogen when it is in its vegetative phase, and then, once it reaches the flowering phase, it will need more potassium and phosphorus.

The majority of macronutrients can be found in a two-part mixture; this is to keep the elements from mixing together and forming an inert solid that you won't be able to use. This means you will have two bottles, bottle 1 and bottle 2, for vegetative growth, and then another two for flowering growth. You will also have a micro-nutrient mixture. Besides these, you may want to have a Cal/Mag supplement. Some cannabis strains are going to have to have more magnesium and calcium than other strains.

Once you have your nutrients, all you are going to do is mix them with some water according to what the packaging says. It is always best to start with a half-strength mixture since marijuana can be burned easily. It tends to be worse on your plants if you overfeed them than underfeed them, and over time, you are going to learn what your plants will need simply by looking at them

You should also have a pH meter on hand so that you are able to easily check the pH level of your water whenever you mix up your nutrients. Cannabis likes to have a pH between six and seven in its soil, and between 5.5 and 6.5 when it comes to their hydroponic media. If the pH gets out of this range, it can end up causing a nutrient lockout, which means that the plants won't be able to absorb the nutrients it is going to need, so make sure that you test the water on a regular basis and make sure that your nutrient mix that you are feeding your plants with is in the range you need.

Watering Your Plants

A lot of people don't even think about what kind of water they use when they are watering their plants. It's easy to think, it is okay for me to drink, why wouldn't it be okay for may plants? For some people, it might not be a problem, but there is some water that contains quite a bit of dissolved minerals. These can build up within the roots of your plants, which will affect how well they are able to absorb their nutrients, or it could contain a fungus or pathogen that doesn't affect humans but can hurt the roots.

Plus, some places will have a lot of chlorine in the water, and this can hurt the helpful microbes in your soil. For this reason, you may want to think about using filtered water.

The main thing you need to remember is to make sure that you don't overwater your cannabis plants. Cannabis can easily develop a fungal root disease if they have to live in too much water, and overwatering is a common mistake that beginners will often make.

How often the plants need to be watered is all going to depend on the type of growing medium you have picked out, the plant size, and the grow room temperature. Some people will wait until the lower leaves on their plants start to droop a bit before they water them.

You need to make sure that, if not using a hydroponic system, the containers you have your plants in are well-draining. Your containers should have holes drilled in the bottom and a container below them to catch the water as it drains off. You want to simply moisten the soil and not saturate it.

As you begin to gain more knowledge and experience, you will start to change up your growing setup and the equipment that you use to fit into your techniques, environment, and what strains you are growing. Keep in mind that growing cannabis is very much a labor of love, so you are going to want to make sure that you give your plants plenty of time.

You may not be able to watch over your plants 24/7, but you can an adequate amount of care by setting aside a few minutes every day. You should have a routine set up where you check on your plants where you make sure that the temperature is right, water and pH levels are correct, and the humidity is just right.

Also, you should also make sure that you keep an eye out for male crops. You are looking to grow high-THC buds, so you have to make sure that all you have in your grow room is female plants. A single male plant can cause huge problems for your garden.

CHAPTER 13

GROWING OUTDOORS: SOIL, FERTILIZERS, AND WATER

— ◆◇◆ —

Growing cannabis can be a very rewarding and fun experience, but it comes with its own challenges and takes some time and money. For the first-time grower without a lot of resources, growing indoors is likely too costly. The great news is that even the smallest outdoor cannabis garden can provide you with lots of great marijuana without the big expense of creating an indoor garden. All you need is a sunny spot, a rooftop, balcony, or terrace, and you can grow cannabis successfully.

Benefits for Outdoor Growing

There are many benefits to growing cannabis outdoors, but the most common reasons are:

- Low Cost – Since you will be relying on the sun, you aren't going to have to spend a bunch of money on grow lights. You may need some soil, clones, seeds, or fertilizer, and possible a small greenhouse to get things started. But you aren't going to need to pay for dehumidifiers, AC units, or electricity for lights.

- Big Yields – When it comes to outdoor plants, the sky's the limit. You can allow them to get as big and tall as you would like, as long they remain manageable. A single plant can yield a pound of weed. Growing just a handful for yourself is plenty. When you grow indoors, your space is a lot more restricted.

- Environmentally Friendly – Growing indoors can be wasteful, uses a bunch of electricity to power the lights, fans, and other tools. The wind and sun are completely free.

- It's Relaxing and Fun – Don't underestimate how therapeutic it is to garden. It's relaxing to spend some time outside, rolling up your sleeves, and getting your hands in the dirt for a bit. Plus, there's nothing better than smoking stuff you grew yourself.

Think About Your Climate

The first thing you need to do before you start growing cannabis outside is to think about the clime of your area. Cannabis adapts fairly well to different conditions, but it can easily be harmed by extremes. When temperatures stay above 86 degrees, it can cause the plants to stop growing, but if temperatures stay under 55, it can damage them and stunt their growth, and possibly kill them.

High winds and a lot of ran can end up causing physical damage to your crops, which will lower your yields. Too much moisture can end up causing powdery mildew and mold, especially during the plant's flowering stage.

Besides weather patterns, you need to have a good understanding of the day length and how it changes through the season. Here's an example, places at 32° N latitude, such as Savannah, have 14 hours of light on the longest day of the year. Places at 47° N, such as Seattle, have 16 hours of daylight on the longest day of the year.

Having a good understanding of the amount of light you are having during the year is important for making your plants transition from their growing period to their flowering period. If you have experience in growing vegetables, those skills will typically translate easily to growing cannabis.

Choosing a Growing Space

Choosing a space to grow your plants is one of the most important decisions you are going to have to make, especially deciding between planting in-ground or in containers.

You need to make sure that your cannabis plants get as much light as they can get, especially during midday because this is the best quality of light. As fall gets closer, your plants aren't going to get as much sun, and this is what will help to move the plants into their flowering phase. Some wind is great for the plants, especially if live somewhere hot. If you live in a place that has a lot of high winds, you should think about planting it close to a windbreak of some kind, such as large shrubbery, wall, or fence.

Finally, you will want to make sure that you have some security and privacy. A lot of people want to conceal their cannabis garden from possible thieves and nosey neighbors. Large shrubs, trees, or tall fences are the best way to do this unless you live in a secluded space. Legal states also require that you keep your cannabis plants concealed from the street.

Some people will grow in containers and have them placed on balconies or even on their roof to help shield their view. You can place a heavy-gauge wire cage around them to keep animals and thieves out. No matter what you choose, think about the size you would like your end plants to be. When cannabis is grown outside, it can get to 12 feet in height, or more, depending on what you allow it to do.

Pick Genetics

The success of your plants is going to greatly depend on the strain you choose because you want one that works for your location and climate. If cannabis is grown a lot where you live, then the odds are in your favor that there are a lot of strains that will grow well there, and some strains could have easily been bred just for your area.

Plants that you grow from seed are more hearty as a young plant than those grown from clones. Seeds can be planted directly in your garden during early spring, even if it is still on the cool side. The biggest issue is there isn't a guarantee of what type of plant you are going to get. If you don't get feminized seeds, you could have male and female plants, which means you are going to have to sex them out to remove the males.

Even if all of your plants are female, each may end up having a different phenotype. To make sure that you have the best version, you need to make sure that you choose its best phenotype, which can end up taking a while. Most beginners will start out using feminized seeds.

Depending on where you live, you could buy a seedling or clone from a dispensary. There are a lot of growers that choose to avoid these options because they don't grow up to be as sturdy as those that are grown from seeds. You could also use auto-flowering seeds. They will start the bloom as soon as they reach maturity no matter the light they are exposed to. You could have a quick-growing crop, or have several harvests during a year using auto-flowering seeds.

The problem with auto-flowering plants is that they are sometimes less potent.

Get Some Soil

Picking out soil for your outside grown plants works a lot like picking out soil for the plants that are grown indoors. The plants need the same type of soil, no matter whether they are grown inside or outside. The only difference is if you choose to grow them in the ground.

If the soil where you live is made up of a lot of clay, it won't drain well and won't hold oxygen. This means you are going to have to amend it a lot. Around a month before you plan on planting your cannabis, dig into the soil where you are going to plant them and add in worm castings, manure, compost, and other decomposed matter. This will provide it more drainage and aeration and will provide your plants with nutrients.

If the soil is sandy, it may be easy to work with and drains well, but it warms up quickly and does not hold nutrients, especially if it rains a lot. You can do the same thing again, but this time you should add in coco coir, peat moss, or compost that will help bind the soil. Adding mulch on top of the soil will help your plants hold onto water and to keep the roots from getting hot. The ideal growing soil is loamy soil. It holds onto nutrients, moisture, and oxygen, and it also drains well. You won't need to amend loamy soil.

Fertilize

We already know that cannabis has to have micro- and macronutrients, mainly phosphorus, potassium, and nitrogen. When it comes to outdoor plants, how you feed them will depend on the soil you use.

If you understand them, and how they work, then you can use commercial fertilizers. The first-time growing will likely want to avoid these, especially long-release granular fertilizers.

You can buy nutrients solutions that are made specifically for marijuana from a grow shop, but they tend to be expensive and can end up damaging your soil's bacteria. They tend to be made up of synthetic mineral salts, and they are meant to be used for indoor growing operations.

Organic fertilization will use the natural microbial life of your soil and will help to minimize any harmful run-off. There are lots of different types of organic and natural fertilizers that you can buy at home and garden stores, such as kelp meal, bat guano, fish meal, bone meal, and blood meal.

Begin with fertilizers that are readily available and inexpensive. Some will end up releasing nutrients quickly, and your plants will easily use them, while others may end up taking months or weeks to release their usable nutrients. If you do this right, you can combine some products together along with your amendments to your soil to make sure that your plants receive the nutrients they need.

Again, testing soil can help this process so that you know exactly what you need to add to your dirt and how much fertilizer you are going to need to use. If you aren't quite sure how much you should use, be a bit conservative with it as you always have the option to top dress if they start to look like they are deficient in nutrients.

Pick Containers

If you find that you don't have great soil, you may decide that planting them in containers is the best option. If there isn't a good place to put your plants straight into the ground, you can use containers and set them wherever you have a good, sunlit area. If you need to, you can also move them throughout the day so that they can be protected from the wind or heat and take advantage of the sun at all times.

When you grow in planters, you are able to use store-bought cannabis fertilizers that you would use if you were growing indoors since you are using premixed soil. This will help to get rid of a lot of the guesswork when it comes to fertilizing

However, plants that you grow in barrels, pots, or buckets will end up being smaller than the ones that get grown in the ground because the container will restrict their root growth. Basically, the size of your pot will help to determine the size your plant will become, although you can grow large plants even if they are kept in smaller containers if you use the right technique.

In general, a five-gallon pot is a great option if you want a medium to small outdoor plant, and a ten-gallon pot or bigger is best for a large plant. Regardless of its size, you are going to want to protect the roots of your plant from getting too hot from the warm weather because pots are able to conduct heat from the sunlight. This can end up limiting the plant's growth, so you should shade them the best you can when the sun is at its highest.

Water

While outdoor-grown cannabis plants have the benefit of using the rain and groundwater, you will likely still need to water your plants frequently, especially during the hottest part of the year. There are some cannabis plants that are able to consume ten gallons of water a day when the weather is the hottest.

Growers in areas that are arid and hot will sometimes dig down and add rocks or clay below their plants to help slow down the water drainage, or they will plant them in shallow depressions that will help the water to runoff and move towards other plants. To improve water retention, you can also add in water-absorbing polymer crystals. Make sure you water deeply first thing in the morning to ensure they have the water they need during the day.

If you live somewhere where it rains a lot, you may have to take a few precautionary steps to improve the drainage as cannabis roots can develop fungal diseases if they become waterlogged. Some of these techniques include:

- Adding perlite, gravel, or clay pebbles to the soil

- Planting in mounds or raised beds

- Digging ditches that direct water away from the plants

Plants grown in windy or hot areas will have to be water more often since winds and high temperatures will force plants to transpire faster. Remember, over-watering is a very common mistake. Water deeply, and then once the top two inches become dry, you can water again. Getting a moisture meter is a good idea.

CHAPTER 14

GROWING OUTDOORS: PREDATORS AND PESTS

— ◆◇◆ —

There are plenty of benefits to growing your marijuana plants outdoors. You have natural lighting, and it is cheaper and efficient. The in-ground root systems will allow for greater expansion, thus creating larger plants. But there are issues with outdoor growing that you don't have to face with indoor growing. Specifically, pests and weather.

In all honesty, pests are easier to control than the weather. You never know what the weather may do. Form a spontaneous hailstorm to heatwaves, you and your plants are at the mercy of Mother Nature.

Protecting Cannabis From Heat

Your plants will let you know when they are experiencing heat stress by folding their leaves into a taco shape in order to conserve their water. If you catch this early enough, the situation can be rectified in order to salvage to plant, though you may still lose some leaves, and pruning may be needed.

When you see the first signs of heat stress, water your plants immediately. You are not just watering to ensure that they have something to drink, but to keep the roots and leaves cool. As long as they haven't been overwatered, the plants will do a lot better when given some water in the morning so that the water can evaporate during the day to keep them cool.

You can also make sure they are planted in an area that is shaded during the hottest part of the day. You can use a shade net for plants that are in the ground, or, if potted, you can simply move the pots. Planting them in groups can give them a bit of shade, just make sure that they get some sun during the day.

Plants in pots need extra root protection because the container they are in can conduct and collect heat. Make sure the planter is kept away from direct sunlight by putting it inside of a larger pot to give it a barrier and make sure you keep them off tile or concrete surfaces.

Protecting Cannabis From Frost and Hail

A surprise frost or storm can create some damage for your plant. Though they are resilient to minor stresses, a hard hailstorm or frost can be nearly impossible to recover from. To protect them, make sure you cover them immediately with some solid object. A trash bin or bucket tends to work well as do cardboard boxes.

Make sure that you weigh them down with something heavy, and secure them to the soil if need be. For a large growing area, place stakes in the ground that are positioned taller than the plants. Then, all you need to do is drape a large tarp over them and secure with some rope. Heavy rainfall may also wash away a lot of soil, so it is a good idea to build up some extra dirt around the base to prevent root exposure. Once all danger has passed, remove the object or structure. You shouldn't leave them in the dark for too long because it can throw off their photoperiod, which can cause stress or hermaphroditic plants.

Pests

The next issue you have to face with outdoor plants are pests. Pests come in all shapes and sizes, and many of them like to attack different areas of the plant's anatomy in different ways. Outdoor gardens are at a greater risk to pest invasions than indoor gardens, mainly because they are exposed to the elements and all of the critters that live nearby.

Sure, there is the conventional route where you apply different chemicals to try to stave off a pest invasion. However, a lot of pesticides out there are unsafe for human consumption and the environment. Plus, you risk contaminating your cannabis with the chemicals. Let's look at a few methods of prevention that you can use to prevent a pest invasion, and to minimize their damage if they do show up.

- Companion Planting

Companion planting is a holistic, and natural way to keep pests away from your garden. This method of pest control has been used by all types of farmers for centuries. Plus, this is a great way to add other plants to your garden to help boost its aesthetic appeal and diversity. What's more, there are some companion plants that can be served for dinner.

The name tells all. The idea of companion planting is to surround your crop with plant allies to help create many different positive effects, like reducing the risk of disease and pests. Monocultures, or gardens with rows upon rows of the same plant, goes against the living ecosystems in nature. When you walk through the woods, you are witnessing what is call a polyculture, or several different plant types growing together. This is how nature wants things to be.

The diversity that occurs within a polyculture helps to increase the biodiversity and forms a habitat that is beneficial for all of the species, which boosts the health and vitality of the system. When you grow cannabis in a polyculture, instead of just cultivating them in complete isolation, you are recreating their natural environment and protecting them from dangers.

Having a polyculture will help to minimize a lot of risks and helps to attract beneficial predatory insects. Companion plants will act as natural pesticides because of the chemicals that they release into the environment.

Some great companion plants are peppermint, basil, coriander, lavender, and Melissa.

The potent and strong aroma of min will confuse the pests, which may help to protect your cannabis. However, mint likes to take over, so you should make sure you plant them in pots. Garlic chives are another strong scented option. They can help to confuse invaders. Plus, mint and garlic chives are great in many dishes.

Nasturtium is often used as a sacrificial crop when used as a companion plant. They lure the insects away from the other plants and take the hit. The flower of these plants will also attract beneficial predatory insects.

- Soil Sterilization

When you sterilize your soil, it will help to get rid of pest risk from the start. There are a lot of pests and pathogens that live within the soil. Sterilizing the material by exposing it to high temps through steam or solar sterilization will kill off most of these possible threats.

- Beneficial Insects

You can introduce beneficial insects into your cannabis garden to help manage pests. These insects will feed off of other insects that want to harm your cannabis. One example of a beneficial insect is the ichneumonids, which is a parasitic wasp. These can help to keep caterpillar numbers down. Caterpillars can create a lot of damage to the exterior and interior of your cannabis.

The female wasp will inject their eggs into a caterpillar. Once the eggs hatch into larvae, the larvae will eat the caterpillar from the inside. This may not be a pretty picture, but it is very beneficial for the productivity, health, and vitality of your cannabis.

Praying mantis can also be adding to your garden as a beneficial insect. They have a taste for caterpillars, as well as many other bugs. Be careful though. If you have hummingbirds that you like, you may want to limit praying mantis because they will kill hummingbirds.

- Diatomaceous Earth

Diatomaceous earth is basically made up of microscopic shards of fossils that inflict damage on insects that come in contact with it. This can be used as a protective measure to fight against ground dwellers, like ants.

- Neem Oil

The majority of pests, like aphids, are not big fans of neem oil. A simple concoction of neem oil and water added to a mister and sprayed onto your plants can help to deal with numerous invaders.

- Sticky Pads

You can place sticky pads around your cannabis plants to help catch pests that fly through the air. If airborne invaders like gnats land on the pads, they will get stuck.

These pads don't completely get rid of pest problems, but they do help to reduce their numbers

- Netting

So far, we have focused on the tiny bugs. However, there are bigger problems out there that will view your cannabis as a great snack. Birds are high on that list, but there are also large insects that can do much more damage than a bird. Bids shouldn't be much of a problem during the growing cycle. That said, if you plan on letting some plants go to seed, then you should keep a watchful eye out for these winged seed-eaters.

A great way to deter birds from munching on your seeds is to place a net around the perimeter of your crop. Netting works great to keep birds from gaining access to your plants, yet they will also let in beneficial light. Birds at any other time during the growing process can actually be beneficial because they will eat pests like caterpillars.

- Fences

We all love our pets. We wouldn't have them if we didn't, but this unconditional love doesn't keep them from misbehaving and getting into trouble. Dogs and cats love to spend some time outdoors, and they love to explore your garden environments. Some of the most favorite activities tend to be digging holes, pooping, peeing, and running around. While you may be able to train your pets to enjoy the garden space without hurting the plants, a better method may be to place a fence around it so that they can't get in.

CHAPTER 15

BREEDING

— ◆ ◇ ◆ —

A cannabis breeder will usually breed in order to strengthen and purify a strain, combining traits, or improve a certain characteristic such as potency, aromas, higher yields, and other things. When growing and breeding, you need to know exactly where the seeds came from and their genetics. If the breeder of the seed is unable to provide you with a detailed history of how the seeds were bred or what they may have been crossed with, you aren't going to know what you're going to get.

Breeding is a fundamental process of growing cannabis. Most of the time, breeding is done on a commercial scale and is very technical, but as the legalization of marijuana increases, as does the popularity of breeding. You can do it yourself if you want.

Propagation of cannabis tends to be a complicated and lengthy process that will take many years for a person to understand and many more to master. However, a home grower doesn't have to view it as so complicated if they are only looking to breed for their own use. We're going to look at breeding for the home grower.

Why Home Growers Should Breed

Why is breeding cannabis at home such a big deal? For one thing, breeding gives the home grower a chance to grow new hybrids and conserve their current stock. This will help to strengthen and preserve some genetics for future uses. If a home grower has a strain that they like, then breeding is a great way to gain new crops with those genetics.

One the other hand, those who a simply looking to make sure they have seeds for the next year will see breeding as a sustainable choice to keeping those plants growing. Not everybody is going to be able to head back to the seed company or nursery to buy new seeds every year. After all, a single seed can cost more than $20, and a dozen can easily set you back more than $100. For those without a huge budget, breeding could be the only way that they can keep a plant around.

Breeding Basics

A cannabis plant is either male or female. Cannabis consumers tend to be focused on the female plants since they are the ones that produce the buds we all love. But the male plants are important during the breeding process, as they have to pollinate the females.

For example, the Super Lemon Haze strain is a cross, or hybrid, of Lemon Skunk and Super Silver Haze. One day, a grower decided they enjoy some aspects of Lemon

Skunk and some of Super Silver Haze and chose to mix them.

In order to accomplish this, you have to a male of one strain pollinate a female of the other. After the plant gets pollinated, it will produce seeds that contain genetic markers from both plants involved in the pollination. You harvest the seeds and then grow them separately. So which do you pick for each strain, the male or the female?

According to Nat Pennington from Humboldt Seed Company, the female plants tend to carry over more traits than the male. The traits of the male plant, though, tend to be obvious to the experienced grower, so you should make sure that you pick a male plant that is going to complement the traits of the female. That's why the breeding process has to be intentional to be successful.

How Cannabis Is Breed

After the parent strains have been picked out, the male and several females are placed in a breeding chamber together to contain all of the pollen. The breeding chamber can be as basic as an enclosed space with plastic sides, or it can be a specially designed chamber for large-scale breeding.

One male plant is able to pollinate tens of females. This is why you should only have one male plant involved during the pollination process. This process is intentional breeding. Growers who have accidentally grown a male plant amongst their females and it pollinates a crop will understand that a single male plant is able to easily pollinate hundreds of females, filling the entire crop with seeds.

Once the plants are placed in a breeding chamber, you can allow the plants to grow through the vegetative phase for a couple of weeks to let them grow bigger, but you don't have to do that. You can place them in a flowering light cycle of 12/12.

A male will grow pollen sacs once matured, which happens during the first couple of weeks during flowering. Pollen gets released and will land on the female plants as the air moves it. When you have an enclosed breeding space, you can contain the pollen so that you do not have any outside pollination going on.

You can also help this pollination effort by simply shaking the pollen onto the females, or collecting it and applying it directly on the females. The pollinated female plants will continue to grow and flower, and they will grow seeds and buds. The seeds formed will have the genetic makeup of both of the parent plants.

Once the seeds are matured, they will be harvested and stratified. Typically, the harvesting of the flowers will happen three to four weeks before seeds are harvested.

Phenotypes

Most hybrids that you can buy have been put through several breeding rounds to help strengthen the genetics to make sure that the descendants of the hybrid will remain consistent and healthy. Look at it this way. For example, you and your siblings hold different attributes that you got from the same parents. This just like the seeds you produce. Every seed that is created from each round of cross-pollination will have slightly different attributes from their parents. The seeds with various expressions are known as phenotypes.

The plant that creates a set of phenotypes with lots of variety is called heterozygous. When it comes to cannabis, you need to have seeds that are homozygous, which simply means that all of them hold the same genes. Homozygosity keeps the plants producing the same seeds with the same makeup.

Once a strain is crossed, the breeder will have to select the phenotype of the strain that they prefer. With large-scale growers, they want to pick the best phenotype for mass production.

Backcrossing

Things don't stop there. Once a phenotype has been picked out, they will backcross them to help improve their genetics. Backcrossing basically means that you will cross-pollinate with a parent or the new strain itself, simply inbreeding the plant. This will make the strain even homozygous and will help to strengthen all of the desirable traits and helps to ensure those traits will get passed down.

Limitations for the Home Grower

Home growers tend to be limited by space and the number of plants that they are able to grow. This means you can't easily breed several plants at once, but with some forethought and planning, you can work around the issues. You have to adapt to these limitations

Simple Propagation for Home Growers

Despite the roadblocks you may have, this simple propagation technique can be used to help the home grower breed their own seeds.

You are going to need:

- Ties and plastic bags
- Small paintbrush
- Gloves
- Isolated propagation chamber
- A mature female plant at around two to three weeks into the flowering phase
- A mature male cannabis plant at around two to three weeks into the flowering phase – or collected pollen

The first step is to sanitize. You have to make sure that you are working in a sanitized and clean environment. Start by cleaning the isolation chamber for receiving the female plant. This clean space will help to prevent cross-contamination and give you a sanitary and safe place for the plant to mature. Diluting some isopropyl alcohol or bleach into water is good enough. Also, you need to sanitize your pollination tools, such as your paintbrush.

You should make sure that your isolation chamber doesn't have any female plants that you don't want to breed with. This will make sure that you don't have any unwanted cross-pollination. However, if you have more than one female plant that needs to mature in this same space, you can implement some of the following selective pollination techniques.

Next, you will start to collect pollen. The pollen sacs appear during the first couple of weeks into the flowering phase. A little while after that, they will open up, and you will have access to their pollen. After you have picked out the best male plant, make sure that you have it separated from all of your other female plants. You want to collect pollen from the plant without accidentally pollinating a bunch of other female plants.

You should make sure that the male plants are always kept in isolation to make sure that your female plants don't end up getting pollinated when you don't want them to. Through the use of a small paintbrush, you can carefully brush the pollen off into a glass jar or plastic bag.

You have to remember that pollen is "alive," and any type of humidity can affect the pollen's viability. Pollen can be stored in an airtight container and placed in the freezer for a long time. If you know you are going to be using the pollen often, then you may want to keep it stored in the fridge as the change in temperature won't be as drastic as it would from the freezer. Pollen that is properly stored can last for more than a year.

Once the female plant is in bloom, it is mature enough to receive pollen after the flowers start to form a hair-like stigma. The object of this selective pollination is to put the pollen you collected onto a certain branch or cola that you want to produce seeds on. You can get around a hundred seeds from every cola if they are pollinated correctly

Choosing the branch you are going to pollinate is all up to you and what you want to get from the breeding process. One pollinated bud can yield 20 to 30 seeds. To finish up this process:

1. Make sure that you have negative pressure in your isolation chamber before you continue.\

2. Start by getting the container with the pollen, some gloves, and a paintbrush.

3. Gently collect a small portion of the pollen from the bag with the brush. You don't need much because a little goes a long way.

4. Run the brush gently across the female flowers you want to pollination, making sure that you just brush across the tops of the stigmas.

5. Once it has been pollinated, carefully place a bag over it and then tie it off to create a seal. This will keep the pollen from pollinating other colas on the pant. This does not have to be done if you want to pollinate the entire plant in isolation, or

you don't have a problem with finding a few seeds throughout the rest of the plant.

6. To prevent contamination, keep the isolation chamber sealed during the plant's maturation process.

You need to repeat this application process one to three times over the course of a week or two. After the plant has reached its fourth week of flowering, you can quit the application process. If you need to reintroduce the pollinated plant to your grow room with non-pollinated plants, you can rinse it down with a bit of clean water to get rid of excess pollen0. This is not completely fail-proof, but if it is done correctly and carefully, it will help our plant to breathe better.

Seeds are mature once the plant has gone through the entire growing process. You have to make sure that you let your plant go all the way through its life cycle before harvesting the seeds in order to make sure you get the best seeds.

After you harvest and dry your plants, it will be time to collect your seeds. Matured seeds are going to be dark in color and have a striped pattern all over the shell. If you executed this process correctly, you should have a high number of seeds no matter how many colas got pollinated.

For the home grower, the process can simply stop here. You have new seeds to grow more plants with for the following year. Unless you are looking to get into the big leagues, you don't need to worry about picking out a phenotype or backcrossing.

CONCLUSION

— ♦ ◇ ♦ —

Thank you for making it through to the end of the book, let's hope it was informative and able to provide you with all of the tools you need to achieve your goals whatever they may be.

The next step is to pick where you want to grow your plant and start gathering tools you will need. It is important that you have everything you need before you start your growing project because it will go more easily. Make sure that you purchase your items from reputable places. You would hate to find out that your seeds aren't good quality and not have them germinate for you. You have to make sure that you take care of your plants, whether grown inside or outside. Nurture them to make sure that they grow up healthy.

Finally, if you found this book useful in any way, a review on Amazon is always appreciated!

9 781801 097581